Diagnostic Endocrinology

DIAGNOSTIC ENDOCRINOLOGY

SECOND EDITION

PHILIP E. CRYER, M.D.

ASSOCIATE PROFESSOR OF MEDICINE
DIRECTOR, CLINICAL RESEARCH CENTER
WASHINGTON UNIVERSITY SCHOOL OF MEDICINE
AND
ASSOCIATE PHYSICIAN, BARNES HOSPITAL
ST. LOUIS, MISSOURI

New York Oxford
OXFORD UNIVERSITY PRESS
1979

Library of Congress Cataloging in Publication Data

Cryer, Philip E
Diagnostic endocrinology.

Includes bibliographical references and index.
1. Endocrine glands–Diseases–Diagnosis.
2. Clinical endocrinology. I. Title. [DNLM:
1. Diagnosis, laboratory–Methods. 2. Endocrine diseases–Diagnosis.
WK100.3 C957d] RC649.C79 616.4'07'5 78-9938
ISBN 0-19-502525-3 ISBN 0-19-502526-1 pbk.

Printed in the United States of America

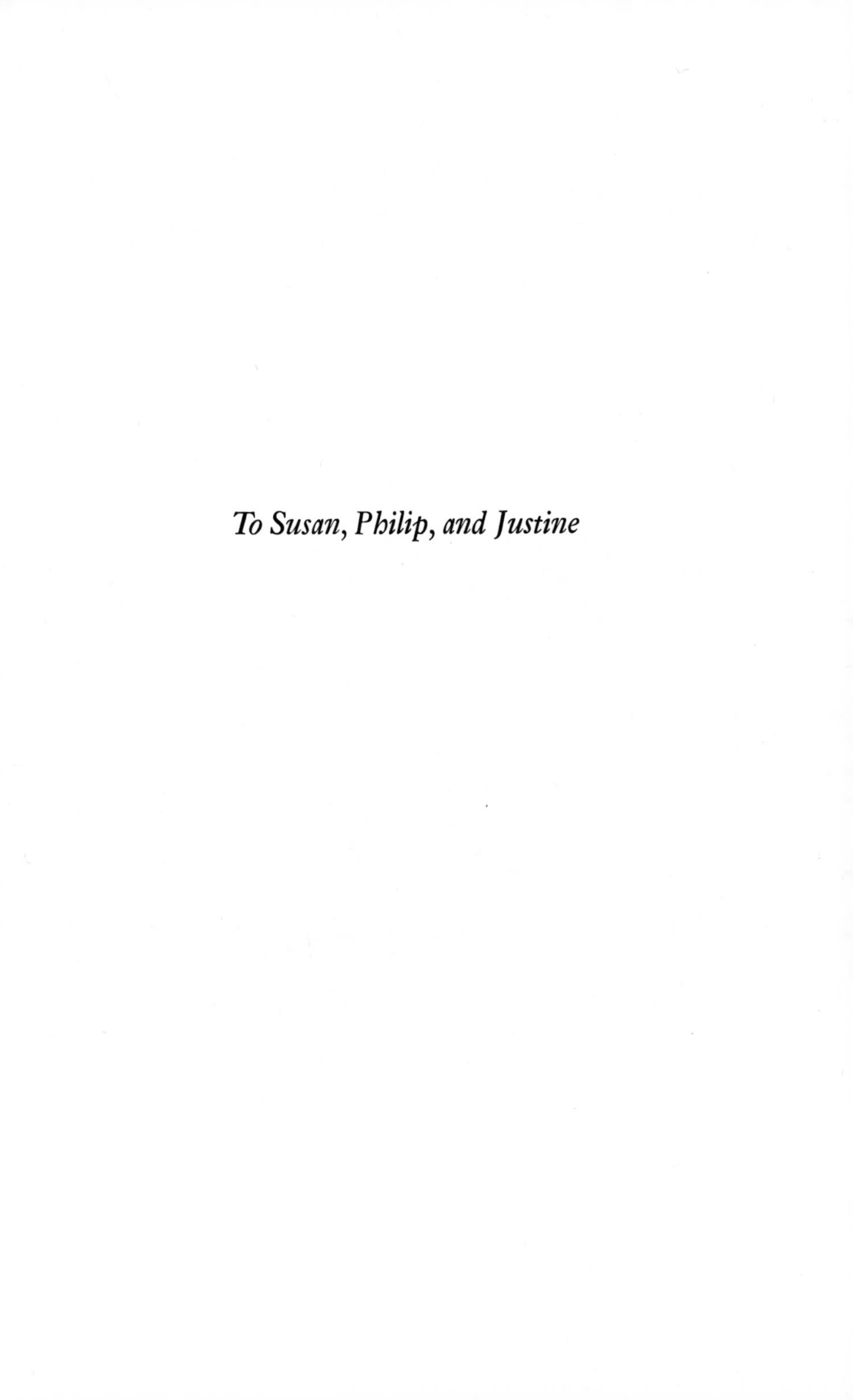

To Susan, Philip, and Justine

PREFACE
to the First Edition

This is not a textbook of endocrinology. Therapeutics have been entirely excluded. Nor is it a treatise on endocrine pathophysiology. In general, after a brief description of normal physiology, aspects of endocrine pathophysiology relevant to diagnosis are discussed. Although clinical features are outlined, the major focus of this book is on the conceptual basis and practical application of modern laboratory methods that are currently available or that will be available in the near future for the diagnosis of functional endocrine disorders. The book is not intended to be comprehensive. Indeed, some traditional diagnostic techniques have been omitted. Rather, the studies discussed represent those judged by the author to be most consistent with efficient, yet conclusive, diagnosis.

This emphasis on biochemical diagnosis is not intended to obscure the critical importance of the clinical evaluation of patients with suspected endocrine disease. Rational selection of hormonal measurements and related diagnostic maneuvers can only be accomplished after careful consideration of the historical and physical findings and any available laboratory data. Furthermore, attempts to interpret "abnormal" hormonal values obtained in the absence of consistent clinical features are often treacherous, although certain endocrine disorders can be diagnosed biochemically before they become clinically apparent.

The author is grateful to several colleagues, including Drs. L. S. Jacobs, L. R. Chase, T. J. Hahn, J. Witztum, G. Schonfeld, A. S. Pagliara, and M. A. Permutt, who read early drafts of various chapters. The critical questions and comments of fellows, house officers, and students have contributed to the content of the book and will, undoubtedly, reveal its shortcomings in the future. Particular gratitude is due Dr. William H. Daughaday for his continued guidance and encouragement. Thanks are also due Ms. Dorothy Turner who typed the manuscript and to Jeffrey House of Oxford University Press for his patience and professionalism.

May 1975 PEC

Washington University School of Medicine
St. Louis, Missouri

PREFACE
to the Second Edition

The acceptance of the first edition of this book has been gratifying. Nonetheless, in view of the accumulation of new information and the ongoing evolution of my approach to the diagnosis of endocrinologic disease, the time has come for updating and revising. The objectives and focus have not been changed in this second edition, although the entire book has been updated and several sections have been rewritten with changes in detail, emphasis, or both.

I am grateful for the comments and questions of many colleagues. Special thanks are due Ms. Doris Brown, for her secretarial assistance, and Mr. Jeffrey House and the staff of Oxford University Press.

July 1978 PEC
Washington University School of Medicine
St. Louis, Missouri

CONTENTS

Diagnostic Endocrinology

INTRODUCTION

COMPETITIVE BINDING ANALYSIS Radioimmunoassays, and the broader concept of competitive binding analysis, have revolutionized clinical endocrinology. These methods have provided the tools that have allowed investigators to clarify the pathophysiology of diverse endocrinologic disorders and to pose basic questions on the biochemical mechanisms of hormone synthesis, secretion, transport, action, and degradation. At the same time, they have made sophisticated diagnostic tests readily available to all physicians who see patients in whom endocrinologic disorders are suspected.

Competition between labeled and unlabeled hormone for specific binding sites on antibodies to the hormone is the basic principle of *radioimmunoassay*. If the quantities of labeled hormone and antibody are constant, the number of molecules of labeled hormone that bind to antibody is an inverse function of the number of unlabeled hormone molecules added to the system. Thus, the higher the concentration of unlabeled hormone the lesser the degree of binding of labeled hormone, and the lower the concentration of unlabeled hormone the greater the degree of binding of labeled hormone. The basic components of a radioimmunoassay system are:

1. Radioactively labeled hormone (easily measured by counting techniques).

2. An antibody with sufficiently high affinity for the hormone.
3. Unlabeled hormone for use as a standard, preferably, but not necessarily, pure.
4. A method for separating antibody bound hormone from free (unbound) hormone.
5. Serum samples with an unknown concentration of hormone to be measured.

An example of a radioimmunoassay standard curve is given in Fig. 1-1. To a series of tubes containing a constant concentration of labeled hormone and antibody, known quantities of unlabeled standard hormone are added. The higher the concentration of unlabeled standard hormone the lower the ratio of bound to free labeled hormone (B/F ratio). Thus, a standard curve can be constructed. If samples of serum containing unknown concentrations of hormone are added to tubes containing the labeled hormone and antibody, as above, the B/F ratio can be determined and the concentration of hormone in the initial serum samples calculated. In the example shown in Fig. 1-1, an unknown sample produced a B/F ratio of 0.3; from the standard curve this corresponds to 2 units of hormone. If 0.1 ml of serum had been added to the assay tube, the initial serum concentration of hormone would have been 20 units/ml.

Conceptually identical assays have been devised using specific binding sites other than those on antibodies. For example, serum binding proteins (thyroxine binding globulin, corticosteroid binding globulin) have been widely used, and an increasing variety of hormone receptors are being used for similar assays. Thus, the more general term, *competitive binding analysis*, has been applied to assays based upon the radioimmunoassay principle.

An obvious advantage of most radioimmunoassay systems is their great sensitivity. In some assays, hormone concentrations as low as 10^{-12} M have been measured. Nonetheless, in several systems normal serum hormone concentrations are near or under the lower limit of sensitivity.

In general, radioimmunoassays exhibit a high degree of specificity, although cross-reactivity with chemically related molecules

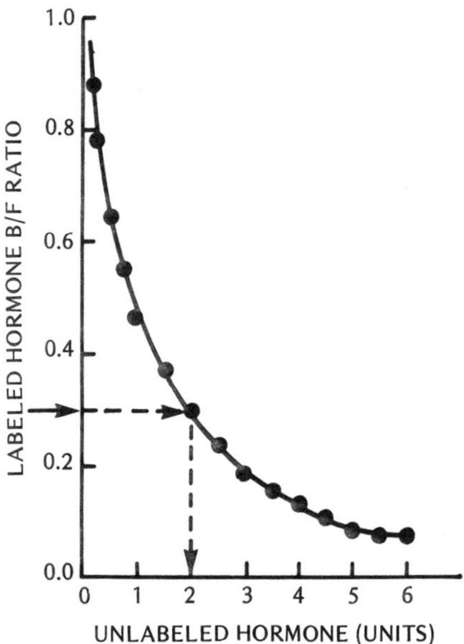

FIG. 1-1. Radioimmunoassay standard curve. If a serum sample containing an unknown hormone concentration yielded a B/F ratio [(antibody) bound to free labeled hormone] of 0.3 (arrow), the quantity of hormone added was 2 units. If the volume of the serum sample added had been 0.1 ml the initial hormone concentration would have been 20 units/ml.

is common. For example, available insulin antiserums cross-react with proinsulin, the insulin precursor. In addition, it is becoming increasingly clear that many peptide hormones circulate in more than one molecular form (precursors, fragments of the parent hormone) and that different antibodies, thought to be raised against the same antigens, may recognize different molecular forms. Although immunoreactive hormone levels generally parallel biologic hormonal activity, it should be emphasized that immunoreactivity and bioactivity are separate characteristics of the hormone molecule. Thus, biologically inactive molecules may be measured by immunoassay. Proinsulin, for example, with less than 10% of the biologic activity of insulin, is measured in insulin radioimmunoassays.

In contrast to sensitivity and specificity, precision is not inherent in radioimmunoassays or competitive binding analysis in general. Thus, every effort to limit experimental error in the laboratory must be made, and serial measurements offer a more solid basis for important clinical decisions than does a single measurement. Additionally, since variation between assays is greater than variation within an assay, it is preferable to measure all samples from a given patient in the same assay. And finally, precision suffers as the limit of assay sensitivity is approached.

As a practical matter, one of the real advantages of radioimmunoassays and related methods is their technical efficiency. After a method has been validated in a given laboratory, 100 samples or more can often be analyzed in a single assay. For the most part, these analyses can be performed economically in hospital and commercial laboratories and be made available to physicians at a relatively low cost to their patients.

It is a basic premise of this book that because of the great clinical utility and relative economy of the sensitive, specific, and sufficiently precise assays based upon competitive binding analysis, hormonal measurements by these methods will become increasingly available to all physicians.

BOUND VERSUS FREE HORMONES In contrast to the polypeptide and glycoprotein hormones, many hormones circulate bound to serum proteins. These include the thyroid hormones, the adrenocortical and gonadal steroids, and vitamin D and related sterols. It is the free (unbound) portion of these hormones that enters the tissues and, therefore, exerts biologic actions and participates in feedback regulation. Thus, it is the free hormone concentration that is biologically and diagnostically relevant. In many instances, measurements of total hormone concentration (bound plus free) provide sufficient diagnostic information. In some instances, however, free hormone concentrations must be measured. Analytic techniques for the measurement of free hormone concentrations are becoming increasingly available.

TARGET ORGAN RESISTANCE TO HORMONES Hormones are, by definition, secreted from glands and transported in the circulation to their target organs. Biologic expression of hormone action requires synthesis and secretion of a biologically active hormone, transport of the hormone to its target organs, interaction of the hormone with cellular receptors in the target organs, and a complex series of intracellular biochemical events ultimately resulting in a characteristic biologic response. Thus, the clinical expression of deficient or excessive hormonal action could result not only from abnormalities in hormone synthesis and secretion (the traditional focus of endocrinologists) but also from the production of abnormal hormone molecules, alterations in the number or affinity of hormone receptors, or abnormalities in the intracellular mechanisms that mediate hormonal action. Alterations in the activity of hormone receptors or intracellular effector mechanisms resulting in target organ resistance and clinical disease have been recognized. These include disorders caused by resistance to thyroid hormones, cortisol, testosterone, and parathyroid hormone. Although less well documented, examples of deficient hormonal action due to the production of biologically inactive hormones have also been reported. To date, however, these disorders appear to be rare with the vast majority of instances of deficient hormone action attributable to deficient hormone secretion. The converse, evidence of excessive hormonal action without excessive hormone production, remains largely theoretical. There is, however, evidence that thyroid hormone excess may produce increased numbers of (myocardial) beta-adrenergic receptors, which perhaps explains the "hyperadrenergic" manifestations of thyrotoxicosis on the basis of enhanced responsiveness to catecholamines without increased catecholamine production.

SUGGESTED READING

1. Parker CW: Radioimmunoassay of Biologically Active Compounds. Prentice-Hall, Englewood Cliffs, New Jersey, 1976.
2. Jaffe BM, Behrman HR (eds): Methods of Hormone Radioimmunoassay, Second Edition. Academic Press, New York, 1978.
3. Yalow RS: Radioimmunoassay: A probe for the fine structure of biologic systems. *Science* 200:1236, 1978.

2

THE HYPOTHALAMUS AND PITUITARY

The adenohypophysis and the neurohypophysis are anatomically and functionally distinct endocrine structures, which, in part, share the sella turcica. The posterior pituitary is an extension of the hypothalamic portion of the neurohypophysis and is little more than a storage site for hormone synthesized within the hypothalamus; essentially normal vasopressin secretion occurs in the absence of the posterior lobe. The adenohypophysis synthesizes, stores, and secretes at least six discrete hormones. The polypeptide hormones include growth hormone (GH), prolactin (PRL), and adrenocorticotropin (ACTH); the glycoprotein hormones include, thyrotropin (TSH), luteinizing hormone (LH), and follicle stimulating hormone (FSH). Nonetheless, adenohypophysial hormone secretion is functionally related to the hypothalamus. The secretion of each adenohypophysial hormone is regulated by hypothalamic (hypophysiotropic) hormones. The adenohypophysial hormones and their corresponding hypophysiotropic hormones are listed in Table 2-1.

A major portion of the blood supply to the adenohypophysis is derived from the superior hypophysial arteries (branches of the internal carotid arteries) via the hypothalamus. Terminal arterioles of these arteries form a capillary network in the median eminence region of the hypothalamus. These capillaries form a system of veins, which drain to the adenohypophysis. This hypo-

Table 2-1

Adenohypophysial hormones and the corresponding hypothalamic (hypophysiotropic) hormones that modify their secretion

ADENOHYPOPHYSIAL HORMONES	HYPOTHALAMIC (HYPOPHYSIOTROPIC) HORMONES	
	+	−
Growth hormone (GH) or somatotropin (STH)	GRF[a]	GIF (SRIF, somatostatin)
Prolactin (PRL)	PRF	PIF[a]
Adrenocorticotropin (ACTH)	CRF	
Thyrotropin (TSH)	TRH	−
Luteinizing hormone (LH)	LH-RH	−
Follicle stimulating hormone (FSH)	LH-RH	−

[a] GRF and PIF appear to be the predominant hypothalamic regulators of GH and PRL secretion, respectively. Hypothalamic destruction results in deficient GH secretion but excessive PRL secretion.

thalamic-adenohypophysial portal system transports hypophysiotropic hormones from the median eminence to the anterior pituitary.

The general hypothalamic-adenohypophysial-target gland relationships are outlined in Fig. 2-1.

GROWTH HORMONE The factors known to alter GH secretion are listed in Table 2-2. Perhaps the most clinically relevant are the stimulatory effects of hypoglycemia, hyperaminoacidemia, and L-dopa, the spike following the onset of sleep, and the suppressive effect of hyperglycemia. The changes in adenohypophysial GH secretion produced by changes in plasma levels of metabolic fuels or hormones and in the level of central nervous system inputs listed in Table 2-2 are all believed to be mediated via the hypothalamus and the secretion of GH releasing factor (GRF) or GH inhibiting factor (GIF) into the hypothalamic-adenohypophysial portal system. The latter factor has been isolated, analyzed, and synthesized by Guillemin and colleagues. This synthetic tetra-

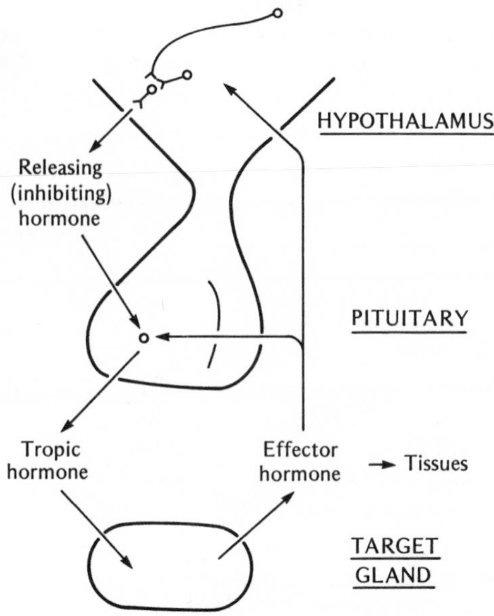

FIG. 2-1. Hypothalamic-adenohypophysial–target gland relationships.

decapeptide inhibits GH secretion in normal subjects and in acromegalics and has been termed somatotropin release inhibiting factor (SRIF) or somatostatin. Somatostatin probably has biologic functions other than inhibition of GH secretion. It has been found in various extra-hypothalamic sites in the brain, gastrointestinal tract, and pancreatic islets and has been shown to suppress the secretion of other hormones including insulin and glucagon.

Dopamine, norepinephrine, and serotonin appear to participate in the hypothalamic regulation of GH secretion. These neurotransmitters are believed to exert their effects via modulation of GRF and GIF secretion from the hypothalamus. Alpha-adrenergic stimulation increases GH secretion; beta-adrenergic stimulation may suppress GH secretion. Dopaminergic stimulation leads to GH secretion in normal subjects (and suppresses GH secretion in acromegalic patients).

Table 2-2

Factors that alter pituitary growth hormone secretion. Various clinical states in which elevated serum GH concentrations have been reported are listed, although their inclusion in one category or another is rather arbitrary and although, in some instances, alterations in GH clearance may contribute to elevated serum levels

	GH SECRETION
Alterations in Metabolic Fuels	
Glucose–Hypoglycemia	Increased
Hyperglycemia	Decreased
Amino acids (e.g., arginine)	Increased
Free fatty acids–Falling	Increased
Rising	Decreased
Prolonged fasting/malnutrition	Increased
Obesity	Decreased
Exercise	Increased
Renal failure	Increased
Hepatic cirrhosis	Increased
Hormonal Effects	
Growth hormone (? via somatomedin)	Decreased
Medroxyprogesterone, glucocorticoids (chronic)	Decreased
Estrogens (chronic, ? decreased somatomedin)	Increased
Glucagon, vasopressin (acute, ? stress)	Increased
Central Nervous System Inputs	
Onset of sleep	Increased
Stress–Surgery/trauma, pyrogen, anxiety	Increased
Emotional deprivation	Decreased (?)
Hypothalamic "maturation" (adolescence)	Increased (?)
Neurotransmitters	
Adrenergic–Alpha	Increased
Beta	Decreased
Serotonergic (5-hydroxytryptamine)	Increased[a]
L-dopa	
Normal subjects	Increased
Acromegalics	Decreased

[a] Recent studies with blocking agents suggest that serotonergic mechanisms may decrease the GH response to sleep and increase the GH response to hypoglycemia.

The major effect of GH is to promote net protein synthesis and tissue growth. It is now clear, at least with respect to cartilage growth, that this effect is not a direct one but is mediated by another hormone, somatomedin (sulfation factor) (SM), which is generated, probably in the liver, in the presence of GH. This factor, or family of factors, may also mediate the negative feedback of GH on GH secretion. The regulation of GH secretion is shown schematically in Fig. 2-2. Growth hormone also impairs glucose utilization, perhaps through intracellular limitation of glucose phosphorylation, an increase in intracellular free fatty acid levels, or both.

It now appears that daily GH secretion varies with age. Somewhat more GH is secreted during the prepubertal and adolescent

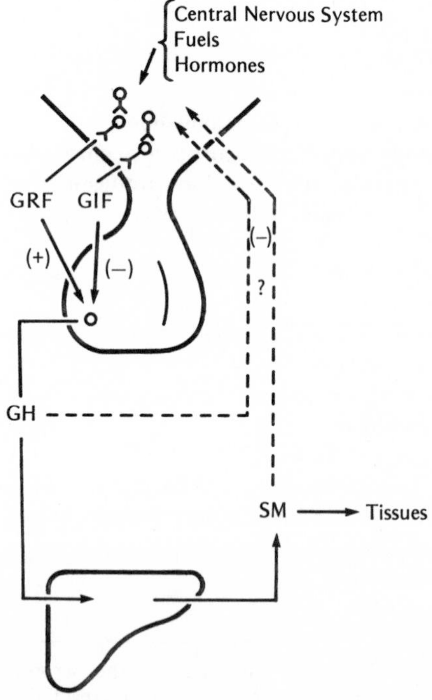

FIG. 2-2. Model of hypothalamic regulation of growth hormone secretion. See Table 2-2 for details.

periods than around middle age. Similarly, GH responses to provocative stimuli, such as L-dopa administration, occur less frequently in older individuals.

PROLACTIN It appears that PRL inhibiting factor (PIF) is the predominant hypothalamic regulator of adenohypophysial PRL secretion. Adrenergic mechanisms also modulate PRL secretion, since catecholamine depleting agents (reserpine, methyldopa) and alpha-adrenergic blocking agents (chlorpromazine) increase PRL secretion, and L-dopa suppresses PRL secretion. In contrast to the control of GH secretion, there is *in vitro* evidence that adrenergic mechanisms may alter the secretion of PRL through a direct effect upon the pituitary (dopamine decreases PRL release *in vitro*). Indeed, it has been suggested that dopamine is PIF.

As with the secretion of GH, PRL secretion increases during sleep, although the PRL peak is considerably less sharp than the GH peak. Stress and exercise trigger PRL release. Increases in serum PRL have been observed during insulin-induced hypoglycemia, but marked hypoglycemia appears to be necessary. The PRL response to infused arginine is relatively minor and at times is not seen. Estrogens stimulate PRL secretion, and this effect is believed to underlie the elevated PRL levels found late in pregnancy. Stimulation of the female breast (e.g., by nursing) triggers an acute increase in PRL secretion.

The only well-established role of PRL in normal human physiology is the stimulation of milk production by the hormonally prepared breast in the female.

THYROTROPIN The secretion of TSH from the anterior pituitary is modulated by a tripeptide hypophysiotropic hormone, thyrotropin releasing hormone (TRH), which has also been synthesized. Thyroid hormones have a negative feedback effect on TSH secretion at the pituitary level. Although TRH is believed to be necessary for normal TSH secretion, its precise role in the regulation of TSH secretion remains to be clarified. Also, TRH is a potent stimulator of PRL secretion.

Various effects of TSH have been observed *in vitro* but the only well-established biologic effect of TSH in humans is the stimulation of thyroid hormone synthesis and secretion.

ADRENOCORTICOTROPIN The secretion of ACTH is modulated by the hypophysiotropic hormone corticotropin releasing factor (CRF), with the pituitary believed to be the major site of negative feedback of cortisol on ACTH secretion. The secretion of CRF is apparently stimulated by neural inputs, including those determining the normal early morning peak in ACTH secretion and the ACTH response to stress. Hypoglycemia also triggers ACTH release, presumably acting through the hypothalamus.

Recent evidence indicates that the material previously identified as melanocyte stimulating hormone (β-MSH), which appears to be secreted in parallel with ACTH, is an extraction artifact. Immunoassays thought to measure β-MSH probably identify a component of a larger molecule (lipotropin) that contains the amino acid sequence of β-MSH. Thus, it remains to be established that β-MSH is secreted as such in man.

Like TSH, ACTH has a variety of *in vitro* effects but its only well-established biologic effect in humans is the stimulation of adrenocortical steroid synthesis and secretion.

LUTEINIZING HORMONE AND FOLLICLE STIMULATING HORMONE The regulation of LH and FSH secretion is complex and, despite recent advances, still poorly understood. A hypothalamic hormone with LH releasing activity (LH-RH or LRF) has been isolated, analyzed, and synthesized. This peptide releases not only LH but also FSH (although its effect on the latter is quantitatively less). Thus, it has been suggested that there is only one gonadotropin releasing hormone for both LH and FSH (LH and FSH have been identified in the same pituitary cell), although the possibility of the existence of a separate FSH releasing hormone has not been excluded.

The feedback control of LH and FSH secretion is incompletely understood. Sex steroids suppress LH secretion presumably through negative feedback at the pituitary level. Although there is negative feedback between spermatogenesis and FSH secretion in men, the mediator involved ("inhibin") has not been identified.

The feedback regulation of FSH secretion in women may also be due to estrogens. At least at high levels, estrogens are believed to exert positive feedback at the hypothalamus. Thus, peak estrogen levels are believed to trigger a mid-cycle burst of LH-RH, which then triggers mid-cycle LH and FSH secretion. The foregoing synthesis must be considered tentative, however; some data have been interpreted as a demonstration of positive feedback at the pituitary. Neural influences on LH-RH secretion are also poorly understood. The effect of emotions on gonadotropin secretion may be mediated through changes in LH-RH secretion, but this remains to be established.

The gonadotropins stimulate gonadal hormone production and gametogenesis.

VASOPRESSIN Arginine vasopressin (AVP, antidiuretic hormone, ADH) is synthesized in neurons of the supraoptic nuclei and transported down axons of these neurohypophysial cells to the posterior pituitary where it is stored before release into the circulation. The secretion of vasopressin depends on the plasma osmolality as monitored by hypothalamic neurons. An increase in plasma osmolality of only a few milliosmoles per kilogram triggers vasopressin release, whereas a small decrease in osmolality suppresses vasopressin release. Major intravascular volume contraction stimulates vasopressin release regardless of plasma tonicity. Central mechanisms, such as severe stress (e.g., surgery), effect vasopressin release. Drugs also alter vasopressin secretion (i.e., alcohol inhibits and narcotic analgesics stimulate release).

Vasopressin increases water resorption from the renal collecting ducts. Thus, with normal renal function, urinary osmolality rises to approximately 1200 mOsm/kg in the presence of maximal levels of vasopressin and falls to approximately 50 mOsm/kg in the absence of vasopressin.

ANALYTICAL METHODS

Radioimmunoassays have been developed for the measurement of all pituitary hormones of recognized biologic importance. These assays have greatly simplified the clinical evaluation of pituitary function. But, certain limitations should be kept in mind. First, the lower limit of sensitivity of many of these assays is currently within the normal range. It is not unusual for normal persons to have unmeasurably low serum levels of GH or TSH. Clearly, such values do not imply deficient secretion of these hormones. Either provocative tests must be performed or the tropic hormone level must be interpreted in light of the level of the target gland hormone. Second, the presence of immunoreactive hormone does not guarantee the presence of biologically active hormone, since the antigenic component of the molecule may be distinct from the biologically active component, and biologically inactive molecules (e.g., prohormones) may be immunologically reactive. These considerations probably explain why different GH antiserums, tested under identical conditions, yield results that vary by as much as 30%.

Radioimmunoassays of GH, TSH, LH, and FSH are generally available. Although the first PRL immunoassay was reported only a few years ago, PRL assays are now performed in many laboratories. The development of radioimmunoassays for ACTH and vasopressin has been particularly difficult, yet ACTH assays are now commercially available. Effective immunoassays for vasopressin have been developed and are becoming increasingly available.

DISORDERS OF HYPOTHALAMIC-PITUITARY FUNCTION

Disorders of pituitary function are summarized as follows.

Hormone	*Deficient Secretion*	*Excessive Secretion*
GH	Short stature	Acromegaly/gigantism
PRL	Failure of lactation	Galactorrhea
ACTH	Adrenocortical insufficiency	Cushing's disease
TSH	Hypothyroidism	Hyperthyroidism (rarely)
LH, FSH	Hypogonadism	—
AVP	Diabetes insipidus	Syndrome of inappropriate ADH secretion

HYPOPITUITARISM

Deficient secretion of anterior pituitary hormones may be due to either disease of the adenohypophysis or disease of the hypothalamus. Deficient vasopressin secretion implies hypothalamic disease, since essentially normal secretion occurs in the (surgical) absence of the posterior lobe of the pituitary. Disordered appetite and temperature regulation, as well as hyperprolactinemia (in the presence of deficiencies of other adenohypophysial hormones and in the absence of a pituitary tumor), also favor a diagnosis of hypothalamic disease.

Isolated deficiency of a single pituitary hormone not infrequently remains unexplained despite thorough diagnostic evaluation. Multiple pituitary hormone deficiencies ("panhypopituitarism") are more often due to pituitary or hypothalamic tumors, pituitary infarction (especially Sheehan's syndrome), or therapeutic pituitary ablation, but unexplained multiple hormone deficiency states are distressingly common. The recognized causes of hypopituitarism are outlined in Table 2-3.

Diagnostic evaluation of a patient with suspected hypopituitarism involves a functional evaluation of the secretory status of the various pituitary hormones and an anatomic evaluation of the hypothalamic and pituitary regions. In the latter evaluation, X-rays of the skull, with views of the sella turcica, and careful ophthalmologic examination, including formal visual field testing, are routinely performed. Conventional laminograms may identify abnormalities of the sella turcica not apparent on plain films. Although there is some dispute about the definitive nature of a negative study, computerized tomographic (CT) scans generally identify suprasellar mass lesions and often delineate the extent of suprasellar extension of masses arising from the sella. Thus, this noninvasive procedure has largely supplanted such invasive procedures as pneumonencephalography and arteriography in the evaluation of parasellar anatomy in many medical centers. The evaluation of a patient with an enlarged sella turcica is discussed later in this chapter.

Table 2-3
Etiologies of hypopituitarism

A. Pituitary
   1. Pituitary tumors (primary, rarely secondary)
   2. Infarction
      a. Postpartum (Sheehan's syndrome)
      b. Arteriosclerotic vascular disease (including carotid aneurysms)
      c. Temporal arteritis, sickle cell disease, cavernous sinus thrombosis
   3. Therapeutic pituitary ablation (surgery, irradiation)
   4. Infiltrative/granulomatous disease–Hemochromatosis, sarcoidosis, histiocytosis, idiopathic granulomatous disease
   5. Infections–Tuberculosis, syphilis, brucellosis, mycoses, etc.
   6. Idiopathic pituitary fibrosis

B. Hypothalamus
   1. Congenital malformations (including hydrocephalus)
   2. Trauma
   3. Tumors–Craniopharyngioma, optic glioma, meningioma, etc.
   4. Infiltrative/granulomatous disease–sarcoidosis, histiocytosis
   5. Infections–Postmeningitis, tuberculosis
   6. Idiopathic (especially, isolated hormone deficiency)

Growth hormone deficiency is suspected in the child with short stature but is not reflected clinically in the otherwise normal adult.* Nonetheless, determination of the capacity to secrete GH is a sensitive test of adenohypophysial function, since GH deficiency occurs relatively early in progressive pituitary disease.

Fewer than 10% of children with heights below the 3rd percentile for their age and sex are found to have deficient GH secretion. Other endocrinologic disorders responsible for short stature in children include delayed puberty, hypothyroidism, and rarely, excessive secretion of glucocorticoids, androgens, or estrogens. Chronic diseases that are primarily non-endocrinologic probably

* The increased insulin sensitivity associated with GH deficiency becomes clinically relevant in diabetic patients receiving exogenous insulin.

are the most common cause of childhood short stature. Clearly, hormonal factors may be involved in such cases. For example, growth retardation with low somatomedin levels despite normal or increased GH levels have been reported in uremic children. Genetic disorders (especially Turner's syndrome) and primary skeletal disorders are less frequently responsible. The remainder may have familial short stature or "constitutional" short stature of unknown etiology.

Basal serum GH levels are usually less than 3 ng/ml and often are below the lower limit of sensitivity of the GH assay. Therefore, provocative tests of GH secretion are usually required to demonstrate normal GH secretion and are always required to document GH deficiency. Three provocative tests–oral L-dopa, intravenous arginine, and insulin-induced hypoglycemia–have been widely used. Normal subjects do not invariably respond to each of these stimuli, and failure to respond to at least two provocative tests is generally required to make a firm diagnosis of GH deficiency. This requirement for unequivocal documentation of deficient GH secretion is particularly important in the child with short stature in view of the limited availability of human GH for therapeutic use.

The L-dopa (L-dihydroxyphenylalanine, levodopa) test is the easiest to perform. After 500 mg of L-dopa (children 30 to 70 pounds, 250 mg; less than 30 pounds, 125 mg) administered orally, with serum samples for GH at −15, 0, 30, 60, 90, and 120 minutes, the serum GH concentration normally peaks between 60 and 120 minutes. Nausea (infrequently with vomiting) commonly follows L-dopa administration, but it is transient. Failure of the GH response to L-dopa has been observed in up to 30% of normal subjects over 50 years old.

Arginine hydrochloride (0.5 gm/kg, 30 gm in most adults) infusion over 30 minutes, with serum samples for GH at −15, 0, 15, 30, 45, 60, 90, and 120 minutes, results in peak GH levels at about 60 minutes. No side effects of intravenous arginine have been recognized aside from the occurrence of hyperkalemia in patients with renal failure.

Insulin-induced hypoglycemia (0.1 units/kg of regular insulin intravenously), with serum samples for GH and glucose at −15, 0, 20, 40, 60, 90, and 120 minutes, produces peak GH levels at approximately 60 minutes. This effective test of GH (and ACTH) secretion can be dangerous and requires the constant attendance of the physician at the bedside. The GH- and ACTH-deficient patient may be insulin sensitive. Some would advocate an initial insulin dose of 0.05 units/kg when these deficiencies are strongly suspected. If insufficient hypoglycemia results, the insulin test can be repeated with 0.1 units of insulin/kg. A fall in plasma glucose to less than 50% of base line after insulin injection is generally required.

Recently, combined provocative stimuli have been advocated. When, for example, oral L-dopa and intravenous arginine are given simultaneously, there is a higher frequency of normal responses than when the two are given separately.

Although an increase in serum GH greater than that attributable to analytical variance after a provocative stimulus indicates that the pituitary can secrete GH, the diagnostic value of these tests can be extended if subnormal, as well as absolutely deficient, responses can be identified. This requires a statistical evaluation of the responses of normal subjects studied with GH assays employing the same antiserum, and thus, normal values must be defined for the specific assay system used. In the GH assay used by the author, peak GH levels over 6 ng/ml are considered normal.

In general, adult women have more brisk GH responses than adult men. Treatment of normal men with stilbestrol, 3 mg daily for 2 days, will increase GH responses to such stimuli as arginine. Also, obese patients (and patients with hypothyroidism) commonly have blunted or even absent GH responses to provocative stimuli.

The measurement of GH 15 to 30 minutes after vigorous exercise (i.e., running up several flights of stairs) has been used as a screening test for GH deficiency in outpatients. But, a single sample 90 minutes after the ingestion of L-dopa has proven effective as a screening test and is probably preferable.

Growth hormone responses to provocative stimuli are illustrated in Fig. 2-3.

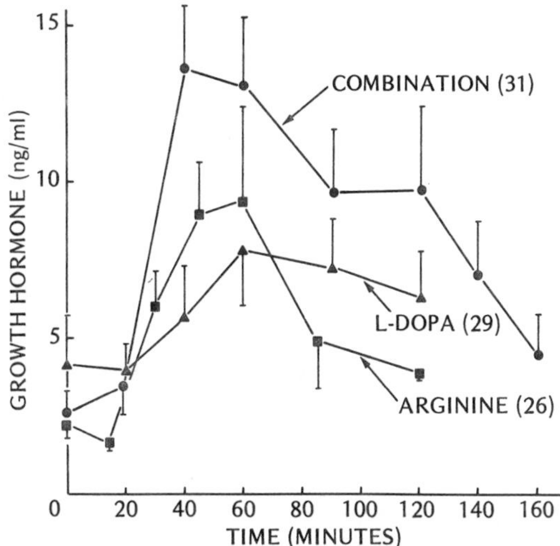

FIG. 2-3. Changes in serum growth hormone (mean ± S.E.) after L-dopa and arginine. (From V. V. Weldon et al: *J Pediatr* 87:540, 1975.)

Deficient prolactin secretion results in failure of postpartum lactation but is not otherwise seen clinically. It is at times difficult to distinguish a patient with deficient PRL secretion from one with normal secretion on the basis of a base-line sample, since normal subjects may have base-line values approaching the lower limit of assay sensitivity. A provocative test for PRL secretory capacity using chlorpromazine (0.7 mg/kg, usually 50 mg in adults) intramuscularly, with samples for PRL at −15, 0, 30, 60, 90, 120, 180, and 240 minutes has been proposed. Peak PRL levels are attained about 60 minutes after chlorpromazine administration in normal subjects. Appreciable side effects, including prolonged postural hypotension, may be associated with these doses of chlorpromazine.

Whereas chlorpromazine is thought to stimulate PRL secretion by a hypothalamic effect, TRH is believed to stimulate PRL secretion by a direct effect on the adenohypophysis. Thus, the TRH test (400 μg of TRH intravenously), with samples at −15, 0, 10, 15, 20, 30, 45, 60, 90, and 120 minutes, can be used to measure pituitary PRL, as well as TSH, reserve. The PRL response occurs quickly after TRH injection. Peak levels are usually reached in 10 to 20 minutes. Transient nausea and a sensation of warmth may follow TRH injection.

A deficient PRL response to TRH is good evidence of pituitary disease. In a patient with evidence of deficiencies of other pituitary hormones and no evidence of pituitary tumor, the finding of hyperprolactinemia raises the possibility of a hypothalamic disorder (with loss of PIF) underlying the hypopituitarism.

The diagnosis of secondary adrenocortical insufficiency, secondary hypothyroidism, and secondary hypogonadism is discussed in the corresponding chapters of this book. Briefly, if the 0800 plasma cortisol is clearly low in a patient with deficiencies of other pituitary hormones and with clinical features compatible with glucocorticoid lack, the diagnosis of *secondary adrenocortical insufficiency* is often presumed; if other deficiencies are not present, an adrenocortical response to exogenous ACTH must be elicited before isolated ACTH deficiency can be diagnosed. If the 0800 plasma cortisol is low normal, partial secondary adrenocortical insufficiency (diminished ACTH reserve) may be present and can be documented by failure of the 0800 plasma 11-deoxycortisol (compound S) level to rise to over 10 μg/100 ml after metyrapone (Metopirone), 750 mg administered orally, every 4 hours for 24 hours. The hypothyroid patient with a low plasma TSH has *secondary hypothyroidism.* Failure of the plasma TSH to respond to intravenous TRH (400 μg) implicates the pituitary, whereas a TSH response to TRH implicates the hypothalamus. Similarly, the hypogonadal patient with a low plasma LH level has *secondary hypogonadism.*

Deficient vasopressin secretion causes *diabetes insipidus.* In many cases, the diagnosis is straightforward. The patient has polyuria (with 24-hour urine volumes of 5 to 10 liters or greater), with corresponding polydipsia and urine osmolalities of 50 to 200 mOsm/kg (specific gravities 1.000 to 1.005); with water restriction, the urine osmolality does not exceed 300 mOsm/kg (1.010). Severe dehydration or incomplete diabetes insipidus may result in urine osmolalities up to 400 mOsm/kg after water deprivation.

Measurement of the osmolality or specific gravity of several first-voided morning urine samples may be of value if the diagnosis of partial diabetes insipidus is considered possible but not likely. A urine osmolality of 800 mOsm/kg (or specific gravity of 1.020) or greater (in the absence of glycosuria or recently injected contrast medium) excludes vasopressin deficiency. If the morning urine is less concentrated, a water deprivation test is indicated.

A water deprivation test should not be undertaken lightly in a patient in whom diabetes insipidus is suspected. The test should be performed early in the day so that the patient can be continuously observed. After base-line measurements of body weight, serum osmolality (or sodium) and urine osmolality, and specific gravity, no water intake is permitted. These measurements should then be repeated hourly. The test should be terminated when the urine osmolality exceeds 800 mOsm/kg (specific gravity 1.020), a normal response, or when more than 3% of body weight is lost. The latter is, in itself, an abnormal response, and the corresponding urine osmolality will be less than 400 mOsm/kg (specific gravity 1.012).

Given an abnormal water deprivation test, it remains to be demonstrated that the kidneys can respond to vasopressin before a firm diagnosis of vasopressin deficiency can be made. This can be accomplished by intravenous infusion of aqueous vasopressin, but the use of a long-acting preparation gives more consistent results. Vasopressin tannate-in-oil (Pitressin tannate), 5 units, is given intramuscularly at 1900 hours. This material must be thoroughly mixed before it is drawn up for injection. Water intake is *not* restricted overnight but is prohibited during the collection of three hourly urine samples the following morning. These urine samples should be concentrated (greater than 800 mOsm/kg in normal subjects and usually substantially greater than 400 mOsm/kg in the patient with vasopressin deficiency) except in the patient with nephrogenic diabetes insipidus (vasopressin resistance).

Differential diagnosis between diabetes insipidus and prolonged primary polydipsia (e.g., psychogenic polydipsia) may be difficult, since in the latter, blunted responses to water deprivation and to vasopressin (presumably due to renal medullary washout) may occur. The psychiatric disturbance is sometimes overt in patients with psychogenic polydipsia, but it may not be. In contrast to diabetes insipidus, primary polydipsia results in urine concentration after water deprivation exceeding that following vasopressin administration. When this is observed, vasopressin secretion is probably normal, the absolute values notwithstanding.

Employing a sensitive radioimmunoassay of plasma vasopressin, Robertson and co-workers have demonstrated a clear-cut distinction between patients with diabetes insipidus and normal subjects, patients with nephrogenic diabetes insipidus, and patients with psychogenic polydipsia, when plasma AVP levels were measured after water deprivation. More widespread availability of such an assay will greatly simplify this differential diagnosis.

HYPERPITUITARISM

Unlike hypopituitarism, hyperpituitarism most often involves a disturbance in the secretion of a single pituitary hormone. The major exception to this generalization is the overproduction of PRL that may be associated with pituitary tumors that produce other hormones, such as GH or ACTH.

Chronic hypersecretion of GH produces *acromegaly*. If excessive GH secretion occurs before puberty, gigantism results. Striking features of acromegaly include bony enlargement and skin and soft tissue changes. Bone changes are most noticeable in the large, broad hands and feet, prominent supraorbital ridges, and protrusion of the mandible (prognathism) (often with spacing of the lower teeth) of the acromegalic. The skin is thickened and often oily, and the subcutaneous tissues are hypertrophic. Headaches and visual field defects suggest suprasellar extension of pituitary tissue. Although the weights of visceral organs are clearly increased in acromegalic patients, disproportionate enlargement of organs, such as the liver and heart, usually indicates an additional disease process. Patients with acromegaly often complain of heat intolerance and excessive perspiration and may describe symptoms referable to such associated medical problems as those listed in Table 2-4.

The etiology of acromegaly is unknown. Although it has been widely believed to represent a primary pituitary neoplastic process, the primary defect may lie in the hypothalamus or in its central connections. Growth hormone hypersecretion and clinical acromegaly corrected by resection of non-pituitary tumors (bronchial carcinoids, pancreatic islet cell tumor) has been reported in a small number of patients. It is suspected, but not proven, that such tumors secrete a GH releasing substance rather than GH itself.

The diagnosis of acromegaly is based upon (a) consistent clinical features, (b) elevated base-line serum GH concentrations, and (c) failure of the serum GH levels to decline normally follow-

Table 2-4
Clinical features of acromegaly

A. Major features
  1. Excessive growth—Bone, soft tissues
  2. Metabolic abnormalities—Heat intolerance, excessive perspiration
  3. Parasellar manifestations—Headache, visual field defects

B. Complications
  1. Degenerative joint disease
  2. Myopathy
  3. Neuropathy
  4. Hypertension
  5. Heart disease
  6. Cerebrovascular disease
  7. ? Pulmonary disease
  8. Glucose intolerance
  9. Hypopituitarism, parasellar catastrophe

C. Associations
  1. Hyperparathyroidism + Functioning pancreatic islet cell tumors + Pituitary tumor = Multiple endocrine neoplasia, type I
  2. Hyperprolactinemia
  3. Hyperthyroidism (rarely)

ing glucose ingestion. Although random serum GH levels are often high enough to be virtually diagnostic of acromegaly, GH levels vary widely in normal subjects; measurements of serum GH after oral glucose are generally advisable in patients with suspected acromegaly, since they provide multiple GH values and will reveal an abnormal response to a suppressive stimulus. In normal subjects, serum GH levels usually fall to less than 3 ng/ml (and often to undetectable levels) 60 minutes after oral glucose administration. Of 50 acromegalic patients evaluated in Daughaday's laboratory, the minimum post-glucose serum GH level exceeded 15 ng/ml in 48 patients, although values as low as 3 ng/ml occurred in the remaining 2 patients.

In general, the correlation between the magnitude of the clinical manifestations and the degree of elevation of serum GH in acromegalic patients is not good. This may reflect a variety of factors, including duration of disease, variations in responsiveness to GH, and/or quantitative dissociation between immunoreactive and biologically active GH. Whatever the explanation, biochemical documentation of the diagnosis of acromegaly is occasionally difficult and may require serial GH sampling. For example, one of the author's patients exhibited clear-cut clinical acromegaly with mean serum GH levels of 8 ng/ml over a 24-hour period and resolution of her soft tissue changes at a 24-hour mean GH value of 4 ng/ml after pituitary irradiation. The assumption that the results of serial GH sampling reflect GH secretion is based upon the observation that metabolic clearance rates of GH are relatively constant in normal and acromegalic patients.

The clearest clinical expression of hyperprolactinemia is *galactorrhea*. But many patients with elevated serum PRL levels do not have galactorrhea, which reflects the complex hormonal interplay required for milk production. Hyperprolactinemia does not, in itself, cause gynecomastia. Amenorrhea, which is often present in hyperprolactinemic women, has also been attributed to PRL excess. Indeed, it appears that hyperprolactinemia is a rather common cause of secondary amenorrhea. Decreased libido has been reported in hyperprolactinemic men in whom galactorrhea is distinctly uncommon despite major hyperprolactinemia.

Excessive prolactin secretion may occur in patients with pituitary tumors. Whether this oversecretion represents primary lactotroph antonomy or primary hypothalamic disease with secondary lactotroph hyperplasia and subsequent tumor formation is unclear. The observation that 24-hour serum PRL profiles in such patients show wide fluctuations comparable to the profiles seen during the physiologic hyperprolactinemia of late pregnancy favors the latter interpretation as does the recent demonstration of the occurrence of human lactotroph hyperplasia by McKeel and Jacobs. Hyperprolactinemia can also result from the ingestion of a variety of drugs (phenothiazines, tricyclic antidepressants, methyldopa, reserpine, oral contraceptives, benzodiazepines, isoniazid), overt hypothalamic disease (trauma, tumor, etc.), and certain endocrinologic disorders, especially hypothyroidism. It has also been associated with the empty sella syndrome (discussed later in this chapter) and has been attributed to uremia or to the presence of tumors of the lung or kidneys in a small number of patients.

Fewer than one-fourth of patients who present with galactorrhea will have radiographic evidence of a pituitary tumor at the time of initial presentation (the combination of amenorrhea and galactorrhea increases this figure to approximately one-third). Roughly one-fourth of such patients will have one of the other recognized causes of galactorrhea and hyperprolactinemia. Thus, nearly one-half of such patients will have "idiopathic" galactorrhea after the initial evaluation. Some of the latter have microadenomas of the pituitary that are too small to produce enlargement of the sella turcica—such have been found during exploratory pituitary surgery or have become radiographically apparent during subsequent reevaluation—but the actual proportion of patients with idiopathic galactorrhea who harbor a pituitary microadenoma is not known.

Galactorrheic patients with radiographically demonstrable pituitary tumors generally have elevated (roughly greater than 25 ng/ml) serum prolactin concentrations. Although tumor patients occasionally have normal prolactin levels and not infrequently have modest hyperprolactinemia, the finding of marked hyperprolactinemia is a distinct clue to the presence of a pituitary tumor. In the experience of Frantz, for example, all galactorrheic patients with serum prolactin levels greater than 300 ng/ml and more than one-half of those with prolactin levels greater than 100 ng/ml had pituitary tumors. Suppressive and provocative tests are not of great value in identifying patients with prolactin secreting pituitary tumors, although tumor patients commonly exhibit a blunted (less than twofold increment) serum prolactin response to provocative stimuli, such as intravenous TRH. Slight to moderate hyperprolactinemia is the rule in patients with idiopathic galactorrhea and amenorrhea, whereas prolactin levels are not infrequently normal in galactorrheic patients with regular menses. Serum prolactin levels range from normal to moderately elevated in patients with other forms of galactorrhea.

Approximately one-third of patients with pituitary tumors and no clinical evidence of pituitary hypersecretion are found to have hyperprolactinemia. Thus, excessive secretion of PRL would appear to be more common than excessive secretion of GH, ACTH, TSH, or the gonadotropins from pituitary tumors, and the frequency of truly nonfunctional pituitary tumors is probably much lower than previously believed.

The diagnosis of Cushing's syndrome due to excessive pituitary ACTH secretion (*Cushing's disease*) is discussed in Chapter 4. Briefly, the failure of low doses of dexamethasone (0.5 mg every 6 hours for 2 days) to suppress the urinary cortisol excretion normally confirms the diagnosis of Cushing's syndrome, and suppression during high doses of dexamethasone (2.0 mg every 6 hours for 2 days) suggests Cushing's disease.

An elevated plasma TSH in a patient with hyperthyroidism indicates *pituitary hyperthyroidism*, a disorder firmly established in a very small number of cases reported in the literature. Thus, in the vast majority of patients with thyrotoxicosis, the plasma TSH level is (approximately) suppressed.

Although not associated with a distinct clinical syndrome, gonadotropin secreting pituitary tumors have also been recognized.

The *syndrome of inappropriate ADH secretion* (SIADH) may

result from ectopic vasopressin secretion (most commonly from a bronchogenic carcinoma) or from inappropriate neurohypophysial vasopressin secretion. The latter can occur in a variety of disorders of the central nervous system (tumor, vascular disease, trauma, infection, subarachnoid hemorrhage, acute intermittent porphyria) or the lungs (tuberculosis, pneumonia) or upon the administration of certain drugs (chlorpropamide, clofibrate, narcotics, barbiturates, diuretics, cyclophosphamide, vincristime). The dilutional hyponatremia of hypothyroidism and of secondary adrenocortical insufficiency resembles SIADH; recent evidence indicates that these hyponatremias are associated with elevated plasma vasopressin levels and are, therefore, examples of SIADH. In some patients with SIADH, no underlying disorder can be discerned.

The diagnosis of SIADH should be suspected in any hyponatremic patient with a disproportionately low serum urea nitrogen (SUN) (often less than 10 mg/100 ml). In the absence of available vasopressin assays, the following biochemical criteria are utilized to diagnose SIADH:

1. Serum hypotonicity (hyponatremia) with urine that is less than maximally dilute. Since, when the glomerular filtration rate (GFR) is not severely reduced, the urine osmolality should be 50 to 100 mOsm/kg in the absence of vasopressin, a higher urine osmolality is taken as presumptive evidence of the presence of vasopressin at the renal tubules. It should be emphasized that the urine need not be persistently hypertonic relative to serum, only less than maximally dilute, in SIADH.

2. Absence of clinical evidence of intravascular volume contraction and persistence of urinary sodium excretion. Major volume contraction is a potent stimulus to vasopressin secretion and will override the suppressive effect of hypotonicity. Although the hyponatremia associated with volume contraction may be due to vasopressin effect on the renal tubules, vasopressin secretion is not "inappropriate" in this circumstance. Persistent urinary sodium excretion is indirect evidence of volume expansion.

3. Normal renal function.

On the basis of available evidence, it is reasonable to anticipate that more widespread availability of sensitive radioimmunoassays of plasma vasopressin will greatly simplify the diagnosis of SIADH in the future.

ENLARGEMENT OF THE SELLA TURCICA

In the evaluation of a patient with sellar enlargement, the following questions should be raised:

1. Is there excessive pituitary hormone secretion? Pituitary tumors commonly hypersecrete PRL or GH; hypersecretion of ACTH, TSH, or gonadotropins also occurs. In most cases, excessive hormone secretion can be excluded clinically. The major exception to this generalization is hyperprolactinemia, which is not uncommonly found in the absence of galactorrhea. If hormone overproduction is suspected clinically, specific studies designed to confirm the diagnosis and establish a therapeutic base line are indicated.

2. Is there deficient pituitary hormone secretion? Careful evaluation of the integrity of pituitary function is particularly important in determining the need for replacement therapy and providing base-line data in patients with pituitary tumors confined to the sella in whom conservative therapy (e.g., conventional external pituitary irradiation) or no immediate therapy is planned or in patients with the empty sella syndrome (see below). Although studies are routinely performed, it could be argued that the need for extensive study of pituitary function is less pressing in patients when more destructive therapy, such as surgical hypophysectomy or heavy particle irradiation, is planned. Obviously, normal preoperative or pre-irradiation function does not guarantee normal function after therapy. Pragmatically, after pituitary hyperfunction is excluded, one could rule out hypothyroidism, maintain the patient on glucocorticoids during stressful diagnostic procedures and through treatment, and then evaluate for hypopituitarism after treatment.

A minimal hypopituitarism workup for patients with sella enlargement might include: (a) GH and PRL levels during an L-dopa test, (b) a serum T_4 and TSH, (c) an 0800 plasma cortisol and a metyrapone test if the former is not clearly normal, (d) an LH level and serum testosterone (male patient) or estradiol (female patient) concentration, and (e) urinary osmolality (or specific gravity) on several first voided morning urine samples.

3. Is the pituitary enlarged, and if so, does it extend beyond the sella turcica? Evaluation of the intrasellar and parasellar anatomy begins with formal visual field testing, skull films with coned down views of the sella, and laminograms of the sella. The latter not infrequently reveal abnormalities not apparent on plain films including anterior, inferior or posterior extension of an intrasellar mass through the walls of the sella. If CT scans convincingly demonstrate the presence of an intrasellar mass and define the degree of suprasellar extension of the mass, the anatomic evaluation is complete. Not infrequently, however, an air study, such as a pneumoencephalogram, is required to define the limits of suprasellar extension or to exclude the empty sella syndrome. The latter is characterized by herniation of the subarachnoid space (through a defect in the diaphragma sella) into the sella and enlargement of the sella with compression of the pituitary. Typically, pituitary function is intact in patients with the empty sella syndrome. Clearly, one would be ill-advised to treat such a patient with pituitary irradiation or ablation.

SUGGESTED READING

1. Daughaday WH: The adenohypophysis. *In* Textbook of Endocrinology, Fifth Edition. Williams RH (ed). Saunders, Philadelphia, 1974, p 31.
2. Leaf A, Coggins CH: The neurohypophysis. *In* Textbook of Endocrinology, Fifth Edition. Williams RH (ed). Saunders, Philadelphia, 1974, p 80.
3. Cryer PE, Daughaday WH: Growth hormone. *In* Clinical Neuroendocrinology. Martini L, Besser GM (eds). Academic Press, New York, 1977, p 243.
4. Chochinov RH, Daughaday WH: Current concepts of somato-

medin and other biologically related growth factors. *Diabetes* 25: 994, 1976.

5. Cohen KL: Endocrine and drug induced interference with pituitary function tests: A review. *Metabolism* 26:1165, 1977.
6. Lin T, Tucci JR: Provocative tests of growth hormone release. A comparison of results with seven stimuli. *Ann Intern Med* 80:464, 1974.
7. Eddy RL, Gilliland PF, Ibarra JD Jr et al: Human growth hormone release. Comparison of provocative test procedures. *Amer J Med* 56:179, 1974.
8. Snyder PJ, Jacobs LS, Rabello MM et al: Diagnostic value of thyrotropin releasing hormone in pituitary and hypothalamic diseases. Assessment of thyrotrophin and prolactin secretion in 100 patients. *Ann Intern Med* 81:751, 1974.
9. Parks JS, Tenore A, Bongiovanni AM, Kirkland RT: Familial hypopituitarism with large sella turcica. *N Engl J Med* 298:698, 1978.
10. Jordan RM, Kendall JW, Kerber CW: The primary empty sella syndrome. *Amer J Med* 62:569, 1977.
11. Thorner MO: Prolactin: Clinical physiology and the significance and management of hyperprolactinemia. *In* Clinical Neuroendocrinology. Martini L, Besser GM (eds). Academic Press, New York, 1977, p 319.
12. Frantz AG: Prolactin. *N Engl J Med* 298:201, 1978.
13. Kleinberg DL, Noel GL, Frantz AG: Galactorrhea: A study of 235 cases, including 48 with pituitary tumors. *N Engl J Med* 296: 589, 1977.
14. Gomez F, Reyes FI, Faiman G: Nonpuerperal galactorrhea and hyperprolactinemia. Clinical findings, endocrine features and therapeutic responses in 56 cases. *Amer J Med* 62:648, 1977.
15. Lachelin GCL, Abu-Fadil S, Yen SSC: Functional delineation of hyperprolactinemic amenorrhea. *J Clin Endocrinol Metab* 44:1163, 1977.
16. Moses AM, Miller M, Streeten DHP: Pathophysiologic and pharmacologic alterations in the release and action of ADH. *Metabolism* 25:697, 1976.
17. Robertson GL, Mahr EA, Athar S, Sinha T: Development and clinical application of a new method for the radioimmunoassay of arginine vasopressin in human plasma. *J Clin Invest* 52:2340, 1973.

3

THE THYROID

The structures of the biologically important thyroid hormones, thyroxine (T_4) and triiodothyronine (T_3), are shown in Fig. 3-1 and the synthesis of T_4 and T_3 from tyrosine in Fig. 3-2. Thyroid hormone synthesis, storage, and release involves at least seven discrete steps, which are outlined diagrammatically in Fig. 3-3. These steps are:

1. Iodide trapping–the concentration of iodide within the follicular cell by an active process against an electrochemical gradient.

2. Organification–the oxidation of iodide and the iodination of tyrosyl residues of thyroglobulin to form monoiodotyrosine (MIT) and diiodotyrosine (DIT).

3. Coupling–the combination of MIT and DIT to form T_3 and the combination of DIT and DIT to form T_4 within the thyroglobulin molecule.

4. Storage–the disposition of thyroglobulin containing iodotyrosines (MIT, DIT) and iodothyronines (T_3, T_4) into the follicular colloid.

5. Proteolysis–the lysis of thyroglobulin to release MIT, DIT, T_3, and T_4 within the follicular cell. Although thyrotropin (TSH) stimulates virtually all phases of thyroid physiology from iodide trapping to T_3/T_4 release, the earliest effect may be upon the translocation of thyroglobulin containing iodotyrosines and

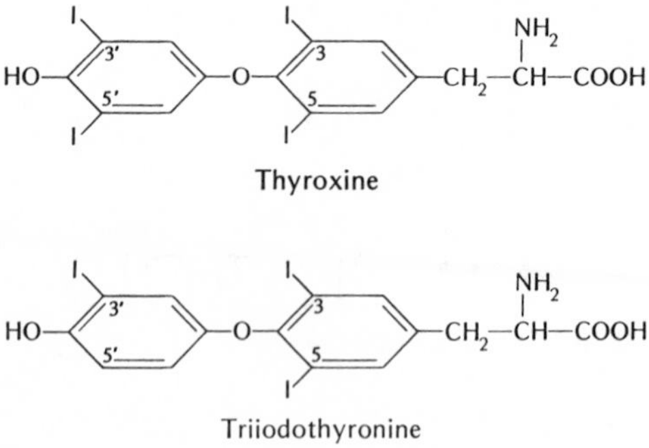

Thyroxine

Triiodothyronine

FIG. 3-1. The structures of thyroxine (T_4) and triiodothyronine (T_3).

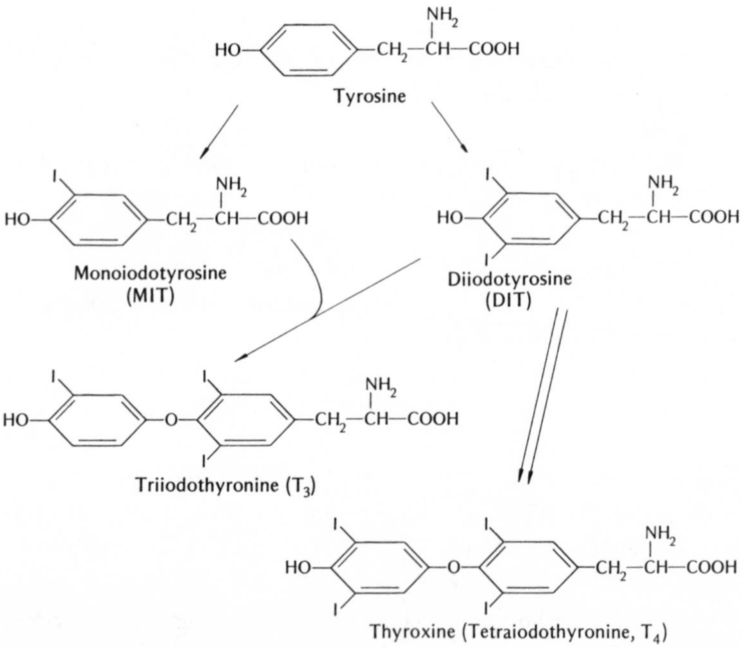

Tyrosine

Monoiodotyrosine (MIT)

Diiodotyrosine (DIT)

Triiodothyronine (T_3)

Thyroxine (Tetraiodothyronine, T_4)

FIG. 3-2. Synthesis of the iodotyrosines (MIT, DIT) and the iodothyronines (T_3, T_4) from tyrosine.

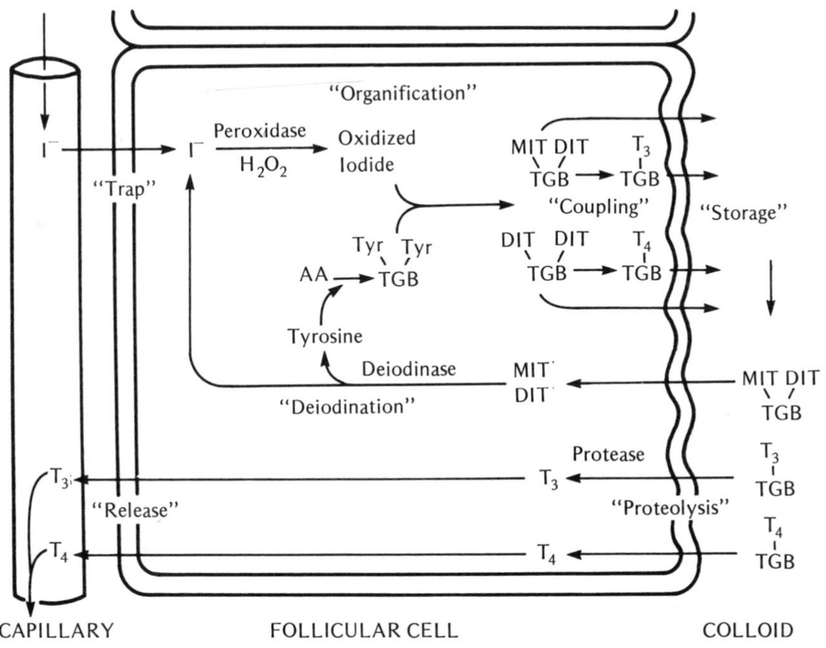

FIG. 3-3. Thyroid hormone synthesis, storage, and release.

iodothyronines from the colloid into the follicular cell where they are exposed to protease activity.

6. Deiodination—the conversion of MIT and DIT to iodide and tyrosine, which can be recycled into thyroid hormones within the follicular cell.

7. Release—the transfer of T_4 and T_3 from the follicular cell into the circulation. Although T_3 is secreted, the predominant secreted product, under normal circumstances, is T_4.

An overview of thyroid hormone physiology is given in Fig. 3-4. Thyroid hormones in the circulation are predominantly bound to serum proteins. Approximately 0.04% of T_4 and 0.4% of T_3 are free (unbound). The rest of the T_4 and T_3 bind to thyroxine binding globulin (TBG, an inter-alpha globulin), thyroxine binding prealbumin (TBPA), and albumin.

Free thyroid hormones are available to the tissues to produce

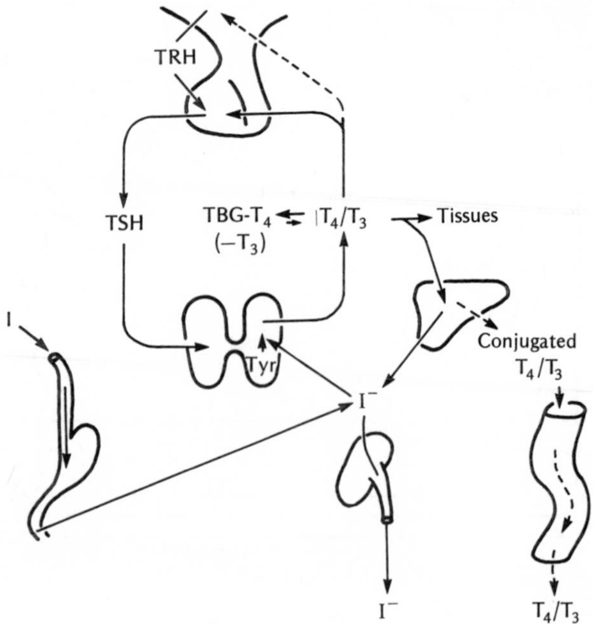

FIG. 3-4. Overview of thyroid physiology.

their typical metabolic effects. Approximately 80% of T_4 is metabolized by deiodination; roughly one-half forms T_3. This, plus the fact that athyreotic subjects treated with synthetic T_4 have essentially normal serum T_3 concentrations, suggests that peripheral conversion from T_4 (rather than thyroidal secretion) is the major source of circulating T_3. Kinetic studies indicate that essentially all of the biologic activity of the thyroid hormones could be attributed to the T_3 generated from T_4; some workers have suggested that T_3 is the biologically active hormone and that T_4 should be considered a prohormone. The finding of euthyroidism in a group of patients with an apparent defect in T_4 to T_3 conversion (the "euthyroid sick") argues against this interpretation, as does the observation that hypothyroid patients made euthyroid by triiodothyronine administration generally have elevated serum T_3 levels.

Although deiodination is the major route of thyroid hormone catabolism, small quantities are conjugated and excreted in the bile. Despite an enterohepatic circulation, small amounts of T_4 and T_3 are excreted in the stool. The hormones also appear intact in the urine in small quantities.

The plasma half-time of T_4 is approximately 7 days, that of T_3 approximately 1.5 days. It would appear that the biologic half-times are considerably longer, since the serum TSH does not rise until 3 to 4 weeks after discontinuation of thyroxine therapy in patients with severe primary hypothyroidism.

The plasma level of free thyroid hormones mediates negative feedback on thyrotropin (TSH) secretion from the anterior pituitary. This negative feedback occurs at the pituitary, rather than the hypothalamic, level. The tripeptide hypothalamic hormone, thyrotropin releasing hormone (TRH), has been synthesized. Thyrotropin releasing hormone stimulates pituitary TSH secretion and its (apparent) absence leads to deficient TSH production.

Thyroid hormones accelerate oxidative metabolism and protein synthesis (in excess they accelerate protein breakdown and cause a net loss of structural protein) through incompletely understood mechanisms. Carbohydrate and fat turnover is increased by thyroid hormones, as is calcium mobilization from bone. Thyroid hormones increase the rate and force of myocardial contraction. Although the old concept that these hormones increase sensitivity to catecholamines has received recent experimental support (T_3 augments the norepinephrine induced increase in the rate of contraction of fetal myocardial cells in tissue culture when it is added at concentrations that have no effect in the absence of norepinephrine and T_3 administration to animals has been reported to increase the number of myocardial β-adrenergic receptors) thyroid hormones have been shown to affect the myocardium directly. Thyroid hormones are critical to normal growth and the maturation of several organ systems, including the brain.

ANALYTICAL METHODS

The major thyroid function tests are listed in Table 3-1. The total serum thyroxine (T_4) concentration is routinely measured by a standard competitive binding technique (Murphy-Pattee) based upon the quantitative displacement of labeled thyroxine from TBG by unlabeled thyroxine (standard or sample) or by radioimmunoassay. An extract of the patient's serum is used in this assay. Thus, the patient's binding proteins are *not* added to the

Table 3-1
Factors that affect the major thyroid function tests

DETERMINATION	METHOD(S)[a]	APPROXIMATE NORMAL VALUES
Thyroxine (T_4)	CBA/RIA	5.0–11.0 μg/100 ml
Triiodothyronine (T_3)	RIA/CBA	0.1–0.2 μg/100 ml
T_3 uptake (T_3U)	(CBA)	35–45%
Thyrotropin (TSH)	RIA	0–8 μU/ml

ALTERATIONS	T_4 (and T_3)	T_3U	TSH	(Free T_4)
Hyperthyroidism	Increased	Increased	Decreased	(Increased)
Hypothyroidism	Decreased	Decreased	Increased or decreased	(Decreased)
Increased TBG	Increased	Decreased	Normal	(Normal)
Estrogens (including pregnancy)				
Acute hepatitis				
Genetic				
Decreased TBG	Decreased	Increased	Normal	(Normal)
Androgens				
Chronic liver disease				
Protein loss (renal, gastrointestinal)				
Genetic				

[a] CBA, competitive binding analysis; RIA, radioimmunoassay.

assay system, and the assay measures total serum thyroxine. The T_3 uptake (T_3U) test is a relatively crude application of the same concept used to estimate the capacity of the patient's serum proteins to bind thyroid hormones (i.e., the number of unoccupied binding sites). The use of labeled T_3 in the T_3U test is merely a technical convenience–the T_3U test does *not* measure serum T_3. In the T_3U test, the patient's whole serum is added to a tube containing labeled T_3, and the fraction of labeled hormone that does not bind to the patient's proteins is determined. If the patient's serum has increased available binding sites (as in hypothyroidism), more labeled T_3 will be distributed to these binding sites, and the T_3U result will be low. If the number of available binding sites is decreased (as in hyperthyroidism), more of the labeled T_3 will be distributed to the resin, and the T_3U result will be high.

The major diagnostic difficulty with the total serum T_4 assay is the distortion introduced by alterations in the levels of endogenous thyroid hormone binding proteins. Elevated TBG levels (during pregnancy; during estrogen therapy, including oral contraceptives; in acute hepatitis; in narcotic addicts or with genetically determined high TBG levels) are associated with elevated total T_4 values. Depressed TBG levels (during androgen or high dose glucocorticoid therapy; in hypoproteinemic states or with genetically determined low TBG levels) are associated with low total T_4 values. In either instance, the concentrations of free thyroid hormones are normal and the patient is euthyroid. Quantitative dialytic estimates of the free T_4 level and measurements of the TBG level are commercially available but are relatively expensive and time-consuming. Thus, the T_3U test is used as an estimate of the binding capacity to detect distortion of the T_4 value by changes in the TBG level. For example, euthyroid estrogen-treated women will have elevated T_4 levels, but since the number of available binding sites is increased, they should have low T_3U values. Conversely, euthyroid nephrotic patients may have low T_4 levels, but since the number of available binding sites is decreased, the T_3U test result should be high.

Thus, the T_3U test should not be viewed as a test of thyroid function but rather as a test of thyroid hormone binding capacity, and it should be used to interpret the corresponding T_4 determinations.

Drugs other than steroids affect thyroid hormone levels. Patients treated chronically with diphenylhydantoin (DPH) often have low serum T_4 (and T_3) levels. Since DPH competitively inhibits T_4 binding to TBG *in vitro*, it has been suggested that the lowered T_4 levels in DPH-treated patients reflect a compensatory decrease in thyroid hormone secretion with the maintenance of a normal free T_4 concentration analogous to the situation in hypoproteinemic patients. Several observations, including the one that T_3U values are generally *not* elevated in DPH-treated patients with low serum T_4 and T_3 levels, suggest that competition is not the sole *in vivo* mechanism. Recent evidence indicates that enhanced metabolic clearance of T_4 and T_3 occurs in DPH-treated patients. It has recently been demonstrated that acetylsalicylic acid also competes with T_4 and T_3 for binding to TBG *in vitro*. In contrast to the observations in DPH-treated patients, free T_4 and T_3 levels are elevated acutely during the ingestion of large doses of aspirin. One might anticipate that patients treated chronically with large doses of aspirin would have low total T_4 and T_3 levels with normal free T_4 and T_3 levels.

A major advance in thyroid diagnosis in recent years has been the development of methods for the measurement of total triiodothyronine (T_3) in serum. Both competitive binding and radioimmunoassay methods for T_3 have been developed. The latter is preferable, and it is commercially available. Alterations in binding activity produce changes in serum T_3 levels qualitatively similar to those in serum T_4 levels.

Serum thyrotropin (TSH), measured by radioimmunoassay, is widely available. With most TSH assays, as many as 30% of euthyroid subjects have unmeasurably low serum TSH levels, since the normal range overlaps the lower limit of assay sensitivity.

The fractional thyroid uptake of ^{131}I is of limited value in the diagnosis of functional disorders of the thyroid, since it is so greatly influenced by iodine intake. It is clear that normal values are considerably lower than previously assumed, probably because of iodine supplementation of foodstuffs. The iodide pool can also be greatly expanded by iodine-containing drugs (especially cough preparations) and by iodinated radiographic contrast materials (bronchograms and myelograms can cause an expanded iodide pool lasting months and years, respectively). Decreased iodide excretion (in renal failure) could produce a qualitatively similar effect. Expansion of the iodide pool results in dilution of the administered ^{131}I and a decrease in the fractional uptake of ^{131}I by the thyroid; absolute thyroidal iodine uptake remains normal, and euthyroidism is maintained. Low fractional ^{131}I uptakes also occur in euthyroid (or transiently hyperthyroid) patients with subacute thyroiditis; the 24-hour value is also suppressed during therapy with antithyroid drugs (propylthiouracil or methimazole). The finding of hyperthyroidism with a low ^{131}I uptake should also raise the possibility of factitious (exogenous) thyrotoxicosis.

On the other hand, elevated fractional ^{131}I uptakes can occur in euthyroid patients with a contracted iodide pool. In the United States, this is rarely due to dietary iodine deficiency but can be produced by combined salt restriction and diuretic administration; it can appear in chronic diarrheal states or the nephrotic syndrome as well. Elevated ^{131}I uptakes also occur in euthyroid or hypothyroid patients with defects in thyroid hormone synthesis (commonly due to Hashimoto's thyroiditis, rarely due to congenital enzymatic defects) and as a rebound phenomenon for several days after discontinuation of antithyroid drug therapy (perhaps reflecting intrathyroidal iodine depletion).

For practical purposes, the ^{131}I uptake is virtually worthless in the diagnosis of hypothyroidism, and many patients with hyperthyroidism have uptake values within the normal range. If the uptake is utilized in the diagnosis of hyperthyroidism a 6-hour, as well as a 24-hour, determination may be of value, since rapid turnover of iodine by the thyroid may result in a misleadingly low 24-hour value in a hyperthyroid patient. The ^{131}I uptake is still routinely used in the estimation of the dose of ^{131}I to be administered therapeutically to patients with hyperthyroidism. Suppression of the ^{131}I uptake serves as an end point in the T_3 suppression test used to demonstrate functional thyroid autonomy, although this test can be performed with serum T_4 as an end point. Since the fetal thyroid concentrates iodine after the 12th week, ^{131}I should not be administered to pregnant patients.

Thyroid scanning is routinely performed with ^{99m}Technetium rather than ^{131}I when an uptake is not being determined simultaneously. The thyroid scan may be one of the most overused endocrine tests. Its value is largely limited to the evaluation of thyroid nodules and the detection of extrathyroidal iodide concentrating tissue (e.g., metastatic carcinoma of the thyroid).

DISORDERS OF THYROID FUNCTION

The major clinical features of excessive or deficient thyroid hormone secretion are listed in Table 3-2. The terms thyrotoxicosis and hyperthyroidism are often used interchangeably, although some investigators use the former for the clinical state caused by excessive circulating thyroid hormones and the latter for those patients with endogenous overproduction of thyroid hormones.

Hyperthyroidism is most often associated with a diffuse goiter (Graves' disease) or with a multinodular goiter (Plummer's disease) or a uninodular goiter (toxic adenoma). Rarely, a diffuse toxic goiter may be caused by excessive pituitary TSH secretion or the ectopic production of a TSH-like material by neoplasms containing chorionic elements. Extrathyroidal production of thyroid hormones (as in struma ovarii) also occurs rarely. Infiltrative ophthalmopathy and pretibial myxedema are manifestations of Graves' disease and are not due to excessive circulating thyroid hormones. Manifestations of ophthalmopathy include proptosis (sometimes with corneal exposure), conjunctival chemosis and injection, extraocular muscle fibrosis, and rarely, loss of visual acuity.

In most instances, the diagnosis of hyperthyroidism is not difficult. The patient has a compatible clinical picture, including a

Table 3-2
Major clinical manifestations of excessive or deficient circulating thyroid hormones

	HYPERTHYROIDISM
Central nervous system stimulation	Hyperkinesis, tremor, hyperreflexia
	Tachycardia/atrial fibrillation
Weight loss	Lid retraction (stare), lid lag
Heat intolerance	Soft skin/fine hair
Weakness	Myopathy
	(Goiter)
	HYPOTHYROIDISM
Central nervous system depression	Hypokinesis, decreased mentation (hypoventilation, coma)
Weight gain	Bradycardia
Cold intolerance	Pseudomyotonia (delayed relaxation phase of reflexes)
Myalgias	
Constipation	Ptosis
Hoarseness	Dry, coarse skin/hair
Excessive menstruation	Dermal infiltration
	(± Goiter)

goiter, and an elevated serum T_4 (and usually T_3U). If the T_4 and T_3U are normal, the diagnosis of hyperthyroidism is less likely but should not be abandoned if the clinical picture is convincing. It is now clear that an appreciable fraction of patients with hyperthyroidism, perhaps 5%, have overproduction of triiodothyronine (T_3) with elevated serum T_3 levels but normal serum T_4 values (T_3-thyrotoxicosis). Thus, the measurement of serum T_3 is appropriate when clinical suspicion is high but the T_4 is normal. There is little reason to believe that T_3-thyrotoxicosis is a distinct entity. Rather it is part of the broad spectrum of hyperthyroidism. Patients with hyperthyroidism and elevated T_4 levels almost invariably have elevated T_3 levels, and as a group, patients with T_3-thyrotoxicosis have mean T_4 values higher than the mean for normal controls. Now that radioimmunoassay measurements of T_3 are widely available, it could be reasoned that the

T_3 level should be the first test performed when hyperthyroidism is suspected, since virtually all hyperthyroid patients have elevated serum T_3 levels. The few recognized hyperthyroid patients with elevated serum T_4 levels but normal T_3 levels have generally had associated illness believed to result in impaired peripheral conversion of T_4 to T_3. Depressed serum TBG levels are a rare, but recognized cause of normal T_4 (and T_3) values in a thyrotoxic patient. Although this diagnosis may be suggested by an elevated T_3U test, it can be conclusively established only by the quantitative measurement of serum TBG and free T_4 levels. Factitious thyrotoxicosis due to the ingestion of triiodothyronine is usually rather easily recognized, since the T_4 is not only not elevated but is suppressed to low levels.

Not infrequently, the question of thyrotoxicosis is raised in a patient in whom a recognized potential explanation for the elevated T_4 exists (e.g., in an estrogen-treated or a pregnant woman). In such patients, judgments based on the degree of elevation of the T_4 are treacherous. The T_4 is usually elevated only a few micrograms per one hundred milliliters during estrogen therapy, but greater elevations do occur. A frankly low T_3U argues against the diagnosis of hyperthyroidism but the question can be resolved conclusively only by measuring the free T_4 level.

Transient hyperthyroidism can occur in patients with subacute thyroiditis (see below). The syndrome is characterized by a relatively short history of clinical hyperthyroidism, a tender goiter, and a very low ^{131}I uptake; it is self-limited. A clinically similar syndrome without thyroid tenderness ("painless thyroiditis") also occurs.

Provocative or suppressive maneuvers, although an interesting exercise in endocrine physiology, are rarely indicated for the diagnosis of hyperthyroidism. For example, the TSH secretory response to intravenous thyrotropin releasing hormone (TRH) is exquisitely sensitive to inhibition by excessive circulating concentrations of free thyroid hormones. Thus, the normal increase in TSH after TRH administration does not occur in patients with hyperthyroidism. The T_3 suppression test is useful in the diagnosis of "euthyroid Graves' disease" (infiltrative ophthalmopathy or pretibial myxedema in a patient with quantitatively normal but nonsuppressible thyroid function) but should not be ordered for a patient with clinical hyperthyroidism, since it involves exposure to 75 μg of T_3 (Cytomel) daily for approximately 7 days if the ^{131}I uptake is used as an end point or 14 days or longer if the serum T_4 is used as an end point. Furthermore, the failure of the ^{131}I uptake or serum T_4 to be suppressed during T_3 ingestion only establishes functional autonomy of the thyroid, not hyperfunction.

Thyroid storm is a life-threatening clinical syndrome characterized by the symptoms and signs of thyrotoxicosis, fever, and eventual vascular collapse. Although it is often described as an intensification of the thyrotoxic state, thyroid storm is not associated with distinct elevations of the serum T_4 (or T_3) over prestorm values. Indeed, the accelerated heat production that occurs in patients with thyrotoxicosis may be a central feature of the pathogenesis of thyroid storm, since the syndrome is often precipitated by factors that limit heat dissipation (e.g., surgical drapes) or conditions that increase heat generation (e.g., infection). The role of stress-initiated adrenergic discharge in the pathogenesis of thyroid storm is unknown but its cardiovascular effects could be amplified in the thyroid hormone stimulated (? sensitized) thyrotoxic patient. Thus, the diagnosis of thyroid storm is a clinical one. For practical purposes, thyrotoxic patients with high fevers should be managed as if they were in storm.

Hypothyroidism may be caused by intrinsic thyroid disease (primary hypothyroidism) or by deficient TSH secretion (secondary hypothyroidism) due to disease of the anterior pituitary or hypothalamus. Primary hypothyroidism may be due to destruction of the thyroid (as in "spontaneous" hypothyroidism, thyroidectomy, ^{131}I therapy, local irradiation, etc.) or to defective thyroid hormone synthesis (in disease due to genetic enzyme defects, chronic thyroiditis, therapy with such antithyroid drugs as propylthiouracil or methimazole, iodine deficiency, etc.) Patients with underlying, but compensated, thyroid disease are particularly susceptible to iodide-induced inhibition of hormone release, and hypothyroidism can be precipitated by iodide therapy. Similarly, lithium inhibits thyroid hormone release and can produce hypothyroidism.

The presence of a goiter in a hypothyroid patient suggests defective hormone synthesis and makes the diagnosis of primary thyroid disease clinically apparent. Obviously, patients with hypothyroidism due to thyroid destruction will not have a goiter and the distinction between primary and secondary disease requires measurement of the serum TSH level.

Secondary hypothyroidism, due to deficient TSH secretion, may be caused by disease of the pituitary or the hypothalamus (TRH deficiency). With the availability of synthetic TRH, differential diagnosis by functional testing is possible. The TRH test is performed by injecting 400 μg of TRH intravenously and measuring serum TSH levels at −15, 0, 15, 30, 45, 60, 90, and 120 minutes. Failure of the serum TSH to rise after TRH injection in a patient with secondary hypothyroidism indicates pituitary disease, whereas a normal increase in TSH after TRH injection implicates the hypothalamus. Examples of the TRH test results in various forms of hypothyroidism are illustrated in Fig. 3-5.

When hypothyroidism is suspected clinically in a goitrous patient, measurement of the serum T_4 and T_3U is sufficient to confirm or disprove the diagnosis of primary hypothyroidism. On the other hand, when confronted with a suspected hypothyroid patient without goiter, the physician should measure the serum TSH as well as the T_4 and the T_3U. The findings of a low T_4 (and T_3U) and an elevated TSH level confirm the diagnosis of primary hypothyroidism, whereas a low T_4 (and T_3U) and an inappropriately low TSH level indicate secondary hypothyroidism. The latter diagnosis should prompt further evaluation of pituitary function as well as a TRH test to distinguish between pituitary and hypothalamic disease. Since blunted growth hormone and cortisol responses to provocative stimuli, as well as elevated prolactin levels, may occur in hypothyroid patients in the absence of pituitary disease, it is reasonable to defer complete pituitary evaluation until euthyroidism is established with replacement therapy. It is mandatory, however, to exclude major adre-

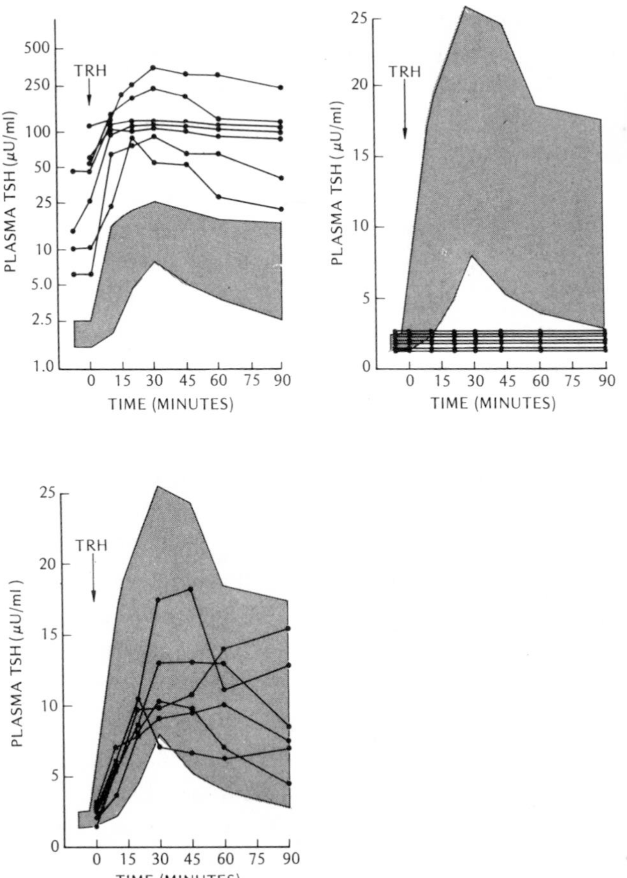

FIG. 3-5. Plasma thyrotropin (TSH) responses to thyrotropin releasing hormone (TRH) in patients with primary hypothyroidism (upper left; note log scale) and with secondary hypothyroidism due to pituitary disease (upper right) or presumed hypothalamic disease (lower left). (From N. Fleischer et al: *J Clin Endocrinol Metab* 35:617, 1972.)

nocortical insufficiency before therapy with thyroid hormone begins, since acute adrenocortical crisis can be precipitated by this therapy if both ACTH and TSH are deficient.*

* An association between primary hypothyroidism and primary adrenocortical insufficiency (Schmidt's syndrome), as well as primary failure of other endocrine glands, has also been recognized.

The anatomic evaluation of the patient with secondary hypothyroidism should include formal visual fields and skull films. It should be recalled that some degree of pituitary enlargement may occur in patients with long-standing primary hypothyroidism. If the sella turcica and visual fields are normal, and there is no clinical evidence of associated hypothalamic disease (diabetes insipidus, abnormalities in appetite or body temperature regulation), invasive procedures (arteriography, pneumoencephalography) are usually not performed in the patient with isolated TSH deficiency. Occasionally, hyperprolactinemia, which is corrected by thyroid hormone replacement, occurs in hypothyroidism. Thus, an elevated serum prolactin level in a patient with secondary hypothyroidism should not be considered collateral evidence of hypothalamic disease unless it persists after adequate thyroid hormone replacement.

So-called "myxedema coma" is the expression of profound hypothyroidism characterized by clinically overt myxedema and severe central nervous system depression with hypoventilation, hypothermia, and stupor proceeding to coma. Once this diagnosis is seriously considered, serum for T_4, T_3U, and TSH levels should be drawn and the patient treated empirically as if both TSH and ACTH deficiencies were present.

Goiter (Table 3-3) may result from hyperplasia of the thyroid follicular cells, infiltration of the thyroid with acute or chronic inflammatory cells, or thyroid cysts or tumors. In the euthyroid or hypothyroid patient, the presence of a diffusely enlarged thyroid most often implies defective thyroid hormone production with a consequent increase in TSH secretion resulting in thyroid hyperplasia. Chronic (Hashimoto's) thyroiditis is a common cause of this type of goiter, which also occurs in a minority of patients treated with iodine or lithium and in patients overtreated with propylthiouracil or methimazole. Congenital enzymatic defects in thyroid hormone synthesis are distinctly uncommon causes of hyperplastic goiter; iodine deficiency, common in other areas, is rare in this country as is the ingestion of goitrogens. The pathogenesis of small, transient goiters that commonly occur during pregnancy and puberty has not been clearly defined but

Table 3-3
Mechanisms and major causes of goiter formation

A. Hyperplasia–TSH (or TSI[a]) dependent; generally diffuse goiters
   1. Euthyroid or hypothyroid patient–Defective thyroid hormone production with consequent increase in TSH secretion
      a. Chronic (Hashimoto's) thyroiditis
      b. Drugs–iodine, lithium, propylthiouracil, methimazole
      c. Enzymatic defects in thyroid hormone synthesis
      d. Iodine deficiency and goitrogen ingestion (rare in U.S.)
      e. Pregnancy
      f. Puberty
   2. Hyperthyroid patient
      a. Graves' disease (TSI dependent)
      b. TSH secreting pituitary tumor (rare)

B. Inflammatory infiltration–Generally diffuse but often asymmetric goiters
      a. Subacute (granulomatous) thyroiditis
      b. Chronic (Hashimoto's) thyroiditis
      c. Riedel's thyroiditis (rare)

C. "Tumors"–Nodular goiters
   1. Benign
      a. Cysts
      b. Adenomas (may produce hyperthyroidism–toxic adenoma or toxic nodular goiter)–Solitary or multiple (multinodular goiter)
   2. Malignant
      a. Primary–Papillary, follicular, medullary, or anaplastic carcinoma
      b. Secondary

[a] TSI = Thyroid stimulating immunoglobulins.

these are reasonably classified as hyperplastic goiters. In hyperthyroid patients, the vast majority of diffuse goiters are a feature of Graves' disease; both goiter formation and hyperthyroidism are thought to be caused by production of thyroid stimulating immunoglobulins in this disease and plasma TSH levels are suppressed. Rarely, a hyperthyroid patient with a diffuse goiter is found to have a TSH secreting pituitary tumor.

In the clinically euthyroid patient with a diffuse goiter, measurements of the serum T_4, T_3U, and TSH are in order. A normal T_4 (and T_3U) confirms the presence of euthyroidism. The finding of an elevated TSH level confirms the suspected pathogenetic sequence and allows the physician to predict that (a) in all likelihood the goiter will continue to enlarge and (b) clinically overt hypothyroidism may develop in the future. Therapy with replacement doses of thyroid hormones is rational in these patients with "compensated hypothyroidism."

The pathogenesis of the common multinodular goiter is unknown. Serum TSH levels and production rates have generally been found to be normal in patients with long-standing multinodular goiters, although one cannot be certain that TSH was not involved early in the course of the disorder. Hypothyroidism, or hyperthyroidism, rarely develops. Although it is common practice among endocrinologists to treat patients with long-standing multinodular goiters with thyroid hormones, it is difficult to see merit in this therapy when the plasma TSH is normal.

The pathogenesis of *thyroid tumors* is also poorly understood. The observations that thyroid tumors develop in experimental animals with drug-induced primary hypothyroidism and do not develop in similar animals in which thyroid hormone has been replaced and that certain malignant thyroid tumors in man clearly regress during thyroid hormone therapy suggest that TSH may be involved in some instances.

Approximately 10% of clinically solitary thyroid nodules are malignant. The capacity of such a nodule to concentrate isotope on scan is good, but not entirely conclusive evidence against the possibility of malignancy.* Such nodules should be followed with the knowledge that they may eventually produce thyrotoxicosis (toxic adenoma). Without histologic examination of the tissue, it is not possible to confidently exclude carcinoma when a solitary

* The observation that a few thyroid cancers concentrate technetium but not ^{131}I may be a reflection of the technique used for the two types of scans. The technetium scan measures early uptake (predominantly trapping), whereas the ^{131}I scan, performed 24 hours after administration of the tracer dose, measures organified ^{131}I.

nodule is isotopically "cold." In the absence of overt evidence of malignancy, little is lost by a few months of observation (with or without "suppressive" doses of thyroid hormones), during which time cysts may regress. Factors that favor prompt surgical excision include a history of childhood irradiation, youth (under 40), the male sex, an unusually hard or irregular nodule or rapid painless enlargement of the nodule, and the finding of stippled calcifications on X-ray films of the neck. Thyroid ultrasonography may be of value in distinguishing solid from cystic thyroid nodules.

It is now apparent that patients who received radiation to the thyroid region in childhood are at particular risk for the development of thyroid carcinoma. Palpable thyroid nodules in such patients should be removed. Palpably normal glands can be followed annually, but it is the author's practice to scan such glands initially, since carcinomas have been found in palpably normal but scan-abnormal thyroid glands in patients with a history of radiation exposure. Lifelong thyroid hormone replacement, on the premise that this may prevent tumor development, and annual follow-up are recommended.

In patients with bilateral pheochromocytomas or pheochromocytoma and hyperparathyroidism, the possibility of associated medullary carcinoma of the thyroid (multiple endocrine neoplasia, type 2) should be considered. This syndrome is often familial. In several instances, medullary carcinoma has been detected in the absence of physical findings by elevated plasma calcitonin levels in members of affected families. The effectiveness of calcitonin measurements in the detection of a suspected medullary carcinoma (e.g., positive family history) in a patient with normal basal calcitonin levels can be enhanced by measuring calcitonin during a calcium infusion (15 mg/kg over 4 hours) or 2 minutes after an intravenous injection of pentagastrin (0.5 μg/kg). Although the results of these tests must be interpreted with a knowledge of the responses of normal subjects with the particular assay used, a several-fold increase in the calcitonin level is highly suggestive of medullary carcinoma.

Thyroiditis is rarely due to pyogenic infection. Subacute

(granulomatous) thyroiditis, thought to be due to viral infection, is not uncommon in outpatient practice. Patients with subacute thyroiditis develop a painful, tender goiter and usually have associated nonspecific symptoms suggestive of viral infection. The course is often prolonged over that of the usual viral infection. When these patients are first seen, the T_4 may be elevated (some patients are transiently thyrotoxic), and the ^{131}I uptake, if performed, is low. Thyroid antibodies are *not* routinely present in the serum. Recently, the occurrence of a clinically similar syndrome without thyroid tenderness (painless thyroiditis) has been emphasized. Patients generally present with hyperthyroidism. Because the hyperthyroidism is transient in this disorder, it is important to distinguish patients with hyperthyroidism due to painless thyroiditis from those with other forms of hyperthyroidism. Thyroiditis with a nontender goiter can be suspected on the basis of a short history of symptoms of hyperthyroidism (and the absence of characteristic features of Graves' disease, such as infiltrative ophthalmopathy or dermopathy) and confirmed by the finding of a very low ^{131}I uptake. It should be recalled that patients with thyrotoxicosis factitia also have low ^{131}I uptakes but do not have goiters.

Chronic (Hashimoto's) thyroiditis most often presents as an asymptomatic goiter. At least 20% of patients with chronic thyroiditis are hypothyroid when first seen. Even when the patient is clinically euthyroid, and the T_4 is normal, it is not uncommon to find the TSH elevated, indicating an impairment in thyroid hormone synthesis. The ^{131}I uptake, if measured, is usually disproportionately high (as it is in other forms of impaired thyroid hormone synthesis). The presence of thyroid antibodies (the thyroid microsomal and thyroglobulin antibodies are often measured) in the serum in high titer is highly suggestive of chronic thyroiditis, although the antibodies may be present in a variety of thyroid disorders and even in the absence of overt thyroid disease. Needle biopsy of the thyroid is routinely used in some centers to confirm the diagnosis of chronic thyroiditis. Often, however, the diagnosis is presumed on clinical, biochemical, and serologic grounds and the patient is treated with thyroid hormone. The coexistence of chronic thyroiditis and Graves' disease has been recognized with increasing frequency, and immunologic similarities between the two diseases have been reported.

Riedel's thyroiditis is rare. The clinical picture is dominated by local compressive symptoms; associated retroperitoneal fibrosis has been recognized. Hypothyroidism occurs occasionally. Thyroid antibodies are not routinely present in the serum.

SUGGESTED READING

1. Werner S, Ingbar S (eds): The Thyroid, Fourt Edition. Harper & Row, Hagerstown, 1978.
2. Ingbar SH, Woeber KA: The thyroid gland. *In* Textbook of Endocrinology, Fifth Edition. Williams RH (ed). Saunders, Philadelphia, 1974, p 95.
3. Stanbury JB: Familial goiter. *In* The Metabolic Basis of Inherited Disease, Fourth Edition, Stanbury JD, Wyngaarden JB, Fredrickson DS (eds). McGraw-Hill, New York, 1978, p 206.
4. Schimmel M, Utiger RD: Thyroidal and peripheral production of thyroid hormones. Review of recent findings and their clinical implications. *Ann Intern Med* 87:760, 1977.
5. Snyder PJ, Jacobs LS, Rabello MM et al: Diagnostic value of thyrotrophin releasing hormone in pituitary and hypothalamic diseases. *Ann Intern Med* 81:751, 1974.
6. Sawin CT, Chopra D, Albano J, Azizi F: The free triiodothyronine (T_3) index. *Ann Intern Med* 88:474, 1978.
7. Birkhauser M, Burer T, Busset R, Burger A: Diagnosis of hyperthyroidism when serum thyroxine alone is raised. *Lancet* 2:53, 1977.
8. Engler D, Donaldson EB, Stockigt JR, Taft P: Hyperthyroidism without triiodothyronine excess: An effect of severe non-thyroidal illness. *J Clin Endocrinol Metab* 46:77, 1978.
9. Shalet SM, Beardwell CG, Lamb AM, Gowland E: Value of routine serum triiodothyronine estimation in diagnosis of thyrotoxicosis. *Lancet* 2:1008, 1975.
10. Davis PJ, Davis FB: Hyperthyroidism in patients over the age of 60 years. *Medicine* 53:161, 1974.
11. Silverstein GE, Burke G, Cogan R: The natural history of the autonomous hyperfunctioning thyroid nodule. *Ann Intern Med* 67:539, 1967.

12. Brown J (moderator): Autoimmune thyroid diseases–Graves' and Hashimoto's. *Ann Intern Med* 88:379, 1978.
13. Greene JN: Subacute thyroiditis. *Amer J Med* 51:97, 1971.
14. Woolf PD: Painless thyroiditis as a cause of hyperthyroidism. *Arch Intern Med* 138:26, 1978.
15. Hennessy JF, Wells SA Jr, Ontjes DA et al: A comparison of pentagastrin injection and calcium infusion as provocative agents for the detection of medullary carcinoma of the thyroid. *J Clin Endocrinol Metab* 39:487, 1974.
16. Schneider AB, Farus MJ, Stachura ME et al: Incidence, prevalence and characteristics of radiation-induced thyroid tumors. *Amer J Med* 64:243, 1978.

4

THE ADRENAL CORTEX

The human adrenal cortex normally produces glucocorticoids (predominantly cortisol), mineralocorticoids (predominantly aldosterone), androgens, and estrogens. Adrenal cortisol and aldosterone secretion are feedback-regulated variables controlled primarily by ACTH and the renin-angiotensin system, respectively. In contrast, sex steroids derived from the adrenal cortex can be viewed as by-products of cortisol synthesis.

The structure of cortisol and certain conventions of steroid nomenclature are illustrated in Fig. 4-1. Figure 4-2 outlines the sequences of steroid biosynthesis. The sequences Δ^5-pregnenolone → progesterone → 17α-hydroxyprogesterone → Δ^4-androstenedione, and Δ^5-pregnenolone → 17α-hydroxypregnenolone → dehydroepiandrosterone (DHA) → Δ^4-androstenedione are common to both the adrenal cortex and the gonads. Although DHA is formed in both the adrenal cortex and the gonads, the bulk of the DHA and its metabolites that enter the circulation (and the urine) are derived from the adrenal cortex, particularly in women. The major sex steroids, testosterone in men and estradiol in women, are primarily derived from direct gonadal secretion. The normal adrenocortical contribution to circulating sex steroid levels is predominantly through peripheral conversion of precursors, such as Δ^4-androstenedione, to sex steroids. Adrenocortical precursors are an important source of the minor sex steroids in the respective sexes—testosterone in women and estradiol in men.

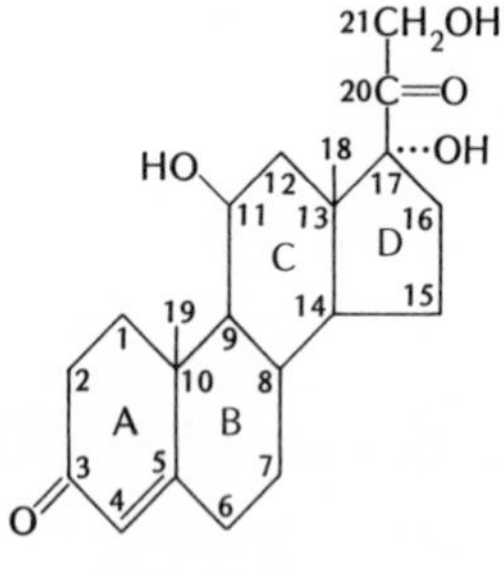

FIG. 4-1. The structure of cortisol and conventions of steroid nomenclature.

In contrast to the pathways common to both the adrenal cortex and the gonads, the biosynthetic sequences from 17α-hydroxyprogesterone to cortisol and from progesterone to aldosterone are limited to the adrenal cortex.

Steroids are sparingly soluble in water and circulate in plasma bound to specific binding proteins and, to a variable degree, to albumin. For example, cortisol binds to corticosteroid binding globulin (CBG), a specific binding protein, which is saturated at plasma cortisol concentrations of approximately 20 μg/100 ml. Thus, free (unbound) cortisol levels increase disproportionately when the total plasma cortisol exceeds this level. Unbound cortisol, the metabolically active component, enters tissues and is filtered and excreted in microgram quantities in the urine. The bulk of secreted cortisol is reduced in the liver to tetrahydrocortisol and cortol (cortisone formed from cortisol is reduced to tetrahydrocortisone and cortolone), as illustrated in Fig. 4-3. These reduced metabolites are conjugated, via the oxygen at C_3, to form the corresponding water-soluble glucuronides that are excreted in the urine in milligram quantities. The secretion and metabolism of cortisol are outlined schematically in Fig. 4-4.

Aldosterone is less avidly bound to plasma proteins than is cortisol. Aldosterone is also reduced and conjugated in the liver and excreted in the urine as tetrahydroaldosterone glucuronide. In addition, approximately 10% of secreted aldosterone is conjugated via the oxygen at C_{18} in the liver and kidneys and excreted as an 18-oxo-glucuronide ("acid labile conjugate").

Clinical disorders characterized by excessive adrenocortical production of all four groups of steroids (glucocorticoids, mineralocorticoids, androgens, and estrogens) have been described. Similarly, deficient adrenal production of glucocorticoids and/or mineralocorticoids produces characteristic clinical syndromes; adrenal androgen lack is clinically recognizable under certain circumstances.

ANALYTICAL METHODS

Although specific methods for the measurement of such steroids as cortisol have been devised, they are generally too complex for routine clinical application. The methods commonly used for the measurement of "cortisol" are not specific but derive relative specificity when cortisol is the predominant steroid in the sample (or extract).

Four nonspecific steroid methods have been used:

1. Colorimetric phenylhydrazine (Porter-Silber) reaction measures steroids with a 17,21-dihydroxy-20-keto side chain (17-hydroxycorticosteroids, 17-OHCS). 11-Deoxycortisol and cortisol and their metabolites are measured.
2. Acid fluorescence measures steroids with an 11-hydroxy group (11-hydroxycorticosteroids, 11-OHCS). Cortisol and corticosterone and their metabolites (plus unidentified steroids and non-steroidal materials) are measured.
3. Competitive binding analysis measures steroids that bind to CBG; these include cortisol, 11-deoxycortisol, corticosterone, and to a lesser extent, 17α-hydroxyprogesterone, 11-deoxycorticosterone, and progesterone.
4. Radioimmunoassay specificities vary, but such assays generally measure steroids other than cortisol, especially 11-deoxycortisol but also 17α-hydroxyprogesterone, corticosterone, 11-deoxycorticosterone, and progesterone.

Competitive binding analysis, based on the displacement of la-

Acetate → Cholesterol → Δ^5 Pregnenolone

Δ^5 Pregnenolone → (C_{17}) → 17α-Hydroxypregnenolone

Δ^5 Pregnenolone → (3βHSD) → Progesterone

17α-Hydroxypregnenolone → Dehydroepiandrosterone (DHA)

17α-Hydroxypregnenolone → (3βHSD) → 17α-Hydroxyprogesterone

Progesterone → (C_{17}) → 17α-Hydroxyprogesterone

Dehydroepiandrosterone (DHA) → (3βHSD) → Δ^4 Androstenedione

17α-Hydroxyprogesterone → Δ^4 Androstenedione

Δ^4 Androstenedione → Testosterone

Δ^4 Androstenedione → Estrone

CH_3 C=O OH HO O

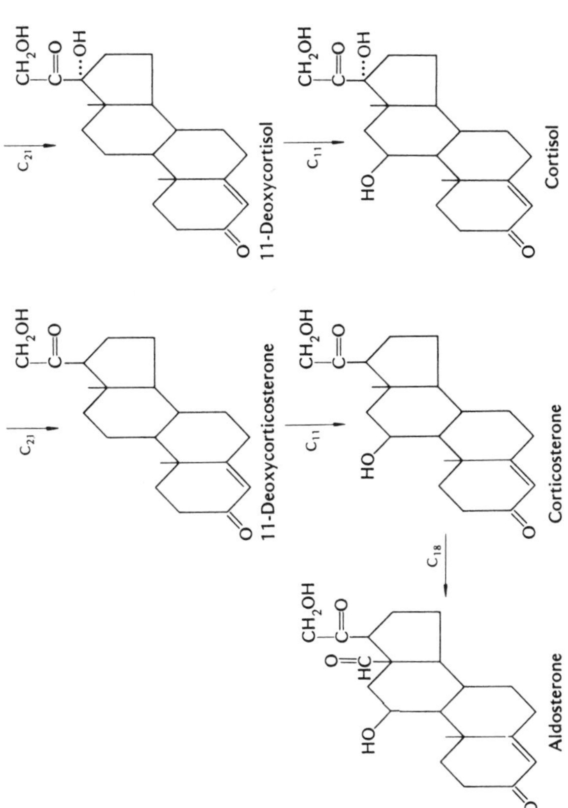

FIG. 4-2. Adrenocortical steroid biosynthesis.

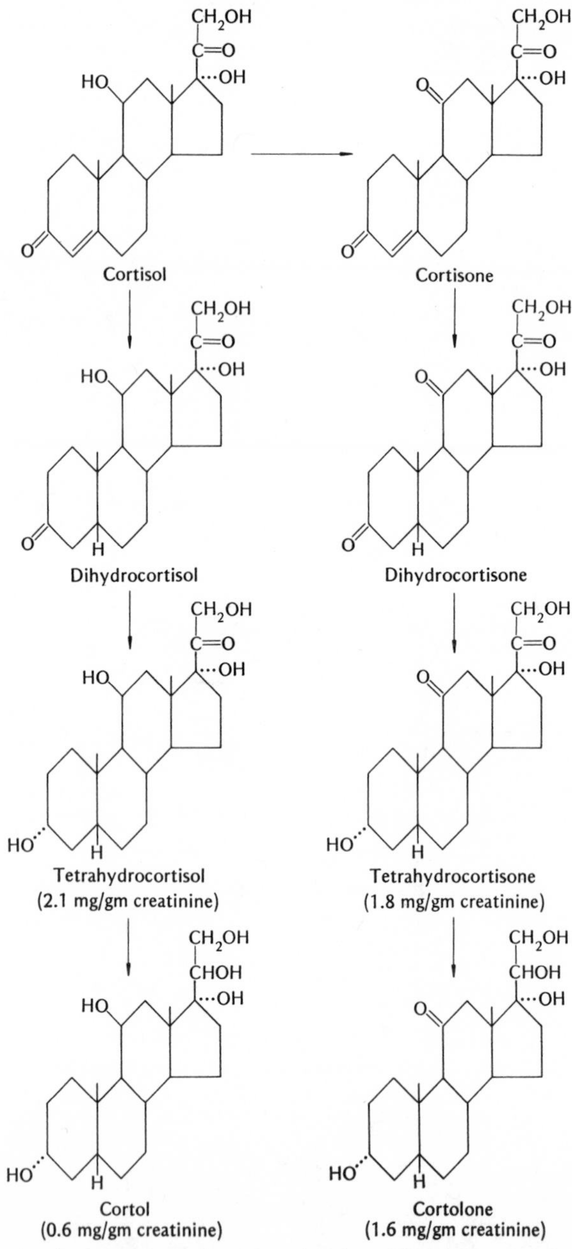

FIG. 4-3. Cortisol (and cortisone) reduction. The values in parentheses represent the approximate daily excretion in normal subjects.

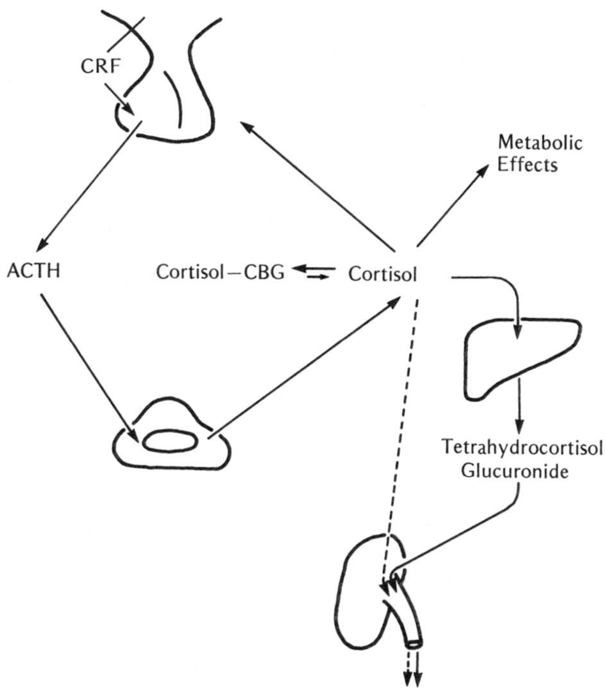

FIG. 4-4. Overview of cortisol secretion, transport, metabolism, and excretion.

beled cortisol from CBG by unlabeled steroid, is often used in the routine measurement of plasma "cortisol." Under most conditions, cortisol is the predominant measured steroid in plasma, and this technique provides a useful estimate of the true cortisol concentration. Under conditions of impaired cortisol synthesis, whether due to adrenocortical disease or to the administration of metyrapone (Metopirone), 11-deoxycortisol or other steroids may be the predominant circulating steroid measured by this method, and the designation "cortisol" is inappropriate. Indeed, the nonspecificity of this method permits the measurement of steroids other than cortisol after selective extraction from plasma. For example, plasma 11-deoxycortisol (compound S) can be measured with the CBG binding system on a benzene extract of plasma (cortisol is not extracted by this solvent). Dexamethasone, a synthetic glucocorticoid, does not cross-react in the competitive binding system. Some degree of cross-reactivity does occur with other synthetic glucocorticoids, such as prednisone and prednisolone.

The competitive binding system can also be used to measure cortisol in urine. The reservations that apply to plasma also apply to urine. Reduced and conjugated cortisol metabolites (the great bulk of the urinary 17-OHCS) are not measured. This determination is designated urinary "free" cortisol; it directly reflects the concentration of free cortisol in the plasma under most circumstances.

Radioimmunoassays for "cortisol" have been developed and applied to plasma and urine. They are becoming more widely available. Given the availability of antiserum, they may provide some technical advantages. But, those assays that have been described to date appear to be no more specific for cortisol than competitive binding systems employing CBG rather than antibody. Slightly lower plasma values have been found with radioimmunoassay in normal subjects.

The colorimetric Porter-Silber determination of urinary 17-hydroxycorticosteroids (17-OHCS) is still used. This technique measures steroids and metabolites possessing a 17,21-dihydroxy-20-keto side chain (11-deoxycortisol and cortisol and their reduced metabolites). The reduced metabolites, such as tetrahydrocortisol and tetrahydrocortisone (Fig. 4-4), are excreted in the urine as glucuronide conjugates. The glucuronide is hydrolyzed, usually with β-glucuronidase, and the resultant unconjugated steroids are extracted with an organic solvent prior to determination. Drugs that competitively inhibit β-glucuronidase, including aspirin in large doses, or that shift the metabolism of cortisol toward the formation of more polar metabolites such as 6β-hydroxycortisol (including phenobarbital, diphenylhydantoin, phenylbutazone, and estrogens) that are not extracted by organic solvents produce artifactually low urinary 17-OHCS. Under ordinary circumstances, the 24-hour urinary 17-OHCS represent approximately 30 to 40% of the daily cortisol secretion. The bulk of the remaining secreted cortisol is excreted as C_{20} reduced metabolites (cortols and cortolones) and other metabolites not measured as Porter-Silber chromogens. Although the Porter-Silber method has served well, in the author's judgment, it should be abandoned in view of the superiority of competitive binding and radioimmunoassay methods for the measurement of cortisol.

Acid fluorescence methods have been used in the past to measure plasma cortisol and urinary "free" cortisol. Due to the large contribution of non-steroidal fluorescence, especially in urine, and to interference by a variety of drugs, fluorometric assays for the measurement of steroids should also be abandoned.

Before the development of competitive binding and radioimmunoassay techniques for the measurement of testosterone, urinary 17-ketosteroids (17-KS), measured colorimetrically (Zimmerman) after acid hydrolysis of the conjugates, were used as an (inadequate) index of androgen secretion. Approximately one-third of urinary 17-KS in men are derived from testicular androgens. The remaining two-thirds in men and virtually all these steroids in women are of adrenocortical origin, derived primarily from dehydroepiandrosterone (DHA) and its reduced metabolites. The 17-KS are notably weak androgens; indeed, androgenic effects of adrenocortical steroids are primarily mediated through the peripheral conversion of DHA and/or androstenedione to testosterone. Nonetheless, the urinary 17-KS are still used as a marker for the adrenocortical component of excessive androgen secretion, particularly in women.

Radioimmunoassay methods for measuring estrone and estradiol in plasma have essentially replaced the less precise chemical methods used to measure urinary estrogens. Radioimmunoassay methods for the measurement of aldosterone in plasma and urine have largely replaced the laborious isotope-derivative methods used in the past.

Urinary steroid determinations, especially with the older chemical methods, are particularly susceptible to error. Although the use of plasma determinations is preferable whenever practicable, urinary measurements provide an integrated reflection of hormone secretion over time and an index of "free" concentrations of hormones that are partially protein bound in the circulation.

"Twenty-four hour" urine collections are all too frequently incomplete often because a physician fails to instruct the nursing staff *and* the patient adequately. Urine collections should be "opened" by having the patient empty his bladder and discard the urine. The urine from all subsequent voidings is saved. The collection is "closed" by having the patient void and save 24 hours after the initial discard. Twenty-four hour urine collections are conventionally opened at 0700 to 0800. This standardized time for opening and closing urine collection reduces the likelihood of collection error and is particularly important for serial collections during suppression and stimulation tests.

The creatinine content should be measured in all 24-hour urine collections. Creatinine excretion is roughly proportional to the lean body mass (men excrete approximately 20 to 25 mg/kg body weight; women excrete approximately 16 to 22 mg/kg body weight), and major collection errors can often be detected from the urinary creatinine content. Perhaps more valuable is the fact that creatinine excretion is relatively constant from day to day in a given individual. Thus, the creatinine content of serial urine collections allows us to estimate the completeness of collection of a given 24-hour urine relative to previous and subsequent urine collections and may prevent errors in the interpretation of suppression or stimulation tests.

Physiologic and pathophysiologic variables hamper the interpretation of urinary steroid determinations. The cortisol secretion rate (and the urinary excretion of cortisol metabolites), for example, is roughly proportional to body mass; large people have higher urinary 17-OHCS than small people, despite comparable plasma cortisol concentrations. Thus, there is considerable overlap in base-line 17-OHCS excretion between obese normal subjects and patients with Cushing's syndrome. Patients with hypothyroidism or liver disease may have impaired cortisol metabolism with low urinary 17-OHCS, and patients with hyperthyroidism may have accelerated cortisol metabolism with elevated urinary 17-OHCS. In either instance, feedback regulation adjusts cortisol secretion, and plasma and urinary cortisol levels are normal.

Alterations in plasma CBG levels affect plasma cortisol concentrations, although the concentration of free cortisol remains normal. For example, plasma cortisol levels are elevated in pregnancy and during estrogen therapy and may be depressed in patients with advanced liver disease or excessive gastrointestinal or renal protein loss. They may also be depressed with androgen therapy. Cortisol excretion should not be affected by changes in plasma CBG levels.*

Drug interference can be a major problem in the evaluation of adrenocortical function. Drugs may alter steroid secretion, metabolism, or excretion, or they may artifactually distort individual analytical techniques (particularly the colorimetric 17-OHCS and 17-KS methods). The effects of drugs on urinary 17-OHCS and 17-KS determinations are summarized in Table 4-1. Clearly, all medications should be avoided during diagnostic study if possible. If medications are absolutely necessary those *known* not to interfere should be selected. If necessary, small doses (including the usual hypnotic doses) of barbiturates can be administered over a few days. Chronic barbiturate therapy, however, results in altered cortisol metabolism and artifactually lowered urinary 17-OHCS. The usual doses of chlordiazepoxide and diazepam do not interfere, at least with short-term administration. Small to moderate doses of ASA or acetaminophen can be used. In contrast, such central nervous system active analgesics as morphine and other narcotics, pentazocine, and even propoxyphene suppress adrenocortical function.

Undoubtedly, factors that influence measurements of other adrenocortical hormones by newer techniques are not yet recognized. An increase in plasma aldosterone occurs with assumption of the upright posture, and a diurnal rhythm, paralleling that of

* Slightly elevated urinary cortisol excretion has been observed in pregnant women by some investigators.

Table 4-1
Effects of some medications on urinary 17-hydroxycorticosteroid (Porter-Silber) and 17-ketosteroid measurements

	17-OHCS	17-KS
Analgesics		
ASA (aspirin) (4 gm/day)	Decreased	0
Acetaminophen	0	0
Phenylbutazone	Decreased	0
Morphine	Decreased	Decreased
Pentazocine	Decreased	Decreased
Propoxyphene	Decreased	Decreased
Phenazopyridine	–	Increased
Tranquilizer–sedatives		
Barbiturates (chronic)	Decreased	0
Chlordiazepoxide	0[a]	0
Diazepam	0	0
Hydroxyzine	Increased	Increased
Meprobamate	Increased	Decreased
Chloral hydrate	0	–
Paraldehyde	Increased	–
Phenaglycodol	0	Increased
Diphenhydramine	0	0
Chlorpromazine	Decreased	Increased
MAO inhibitors	Increased	Increased
Diphenylhydantoin	Decreased	0
Glutethimide	Increased	–
Methyprylon	Increased	Increased
Antihypertensives		
Reserpine	Decreased	Decreased
Hydralazine	0[a]	0
Diuretics		
Thiazides (chronic)	0[a]	0
Thiazides (acute)	Decreased	–
Spironolactone	Increased	Increased
Acetazolamide	0[a]	0
Furosemide (acute)	Decreased	–
Ethacrynic acid (acute)	Decreased	–
Cardiac drugs		
Digoxin	0[a]	0
Digitoxin	0[a]	0
Quinidine	0	0

Table 4-1 Continued

Antimicrobials		
Penicillin (20 million units)	0	Increased
Nalidixic acid	0	Increased
Triacetyloleandomycin	Increased	Increased
Mandelamine	Increased	0
Amphotericin B	Decreased	–
Cloxacillin	Increased	Increased
Miscellaneous		
Estrogens	Decreased	Decreased
Clofibrate	0	Decreased
Probenecid	Decreased	Decreased
Colchicine	Increased	–
Licorice	Increased	–

0, no change.
[a] *In vitro* studies suggest potential interference not confirmed *in vivo.*

cortisol, in plasma aldosterone levels has been described. Factors that affect the levels of sex steroids are discussed in Chapter 5.

DISORDERS OF ADRENOCORTICAL FUNCTION

Clinical disorders of adrenocortical function can be summarized as follows:

Adrenocortical Hyperfunction

		Glucocorticoids	} ← Cushing's syndrome (Glucocorticoids, Mineralocorticoids, Androgens, Estrogens)
Aldosteronism	→	Mineralocorticoids	} ← Enzyme defects in cortisol synthesis (adrenogenital syndromes) (Mineralocorticoids, Androgens)
Virilizing tumors	→	Androgens	
Feminizing tumors	→	Estrogens	

Adrenocortical Hypofunction

Hypopituitarism	→	Glucocorticoids	} Addison's disease
Hypoaldosteronism	→	Mineralocorticoids	
Hypopituitarism	→	Androgens	
		Estrogens	

Table 4-2
Clinical effects of excessive adrenocortical steroids

Glucocorticoids	
Protein catabolism	Thin skin (ecchymoses, striae, plethora) Muscular wasting Osteopenia
Gluconeogenesis	Glucose intolerance
Central nervous system stimulation	Hyperphagia⟶obesity (insomnia, psychosis)
Sodium retention/ catecholamine "sensitization"	Hypertension
Anti-inflammatory	Infections (decreased lymphocytes and eosinophils, increased neutrophils)
Mineralocorticoids	
Sodium retention	Hypertension Hypokalemia
Androgens	
Virilization (women)	Acne Hirsutism Amenorrhea Clitoral enlargement Increased muscle mass Deepened voice Temporal balding
Estrogens	
Feminization (men)	Gynecomastia, decreased testicular size

The clinical effects of excessive and deficient circulating steroids are summarized in Tables 4-2 and 4-3.

GLUCOCORTICOID DISORDERS Excessive circulating glucocorticoids produce *Cushing's syndrome*. As seen clinically, this syndrome is

Table 4-3
Clinical effects of deficient adrenocortical steroids

Glucocorticoids	
Decreased central nervous system stimulation	Weakness, fatigue, lethargy, anorexia⟶weight loss, nausea, vomiting
Decreased catecholamine sensitivity	Hypotension (orthostatic)
Decreased gluconeogenesis	Fasting hypoglycemia
Miscellaneous	Lymphoid hyperplasia, dilutional hyponatremia
Mineralocorticoids	
Sodium loss	Hypotension (orthostatic or absolute), depletional hyponatremia, hyperkalemia, azotemia
Androgens	
Decreased androgen	Decreased pubic/axillary hair (women)

most often due to the administration of excessive quantities of exogenous glucocorticoids in the therapy of non-endocrine disease. Endogenous Cushing's syndrome may be due to an autonomous adrenocortical tumor (adenoma or carcinoma) or tumors, the secretion of an ACTH-like peptide by a nonpituitary tumor (the ectopic ACTH syndrome), or excessive pituitary ACTH secretion (Cushing's disease). Excessive mineralocorticoid and androgen production may occur in the latter disorders, but cortisol overproduction is the hallmark of Cushing's syndrome and the critical diagnostic feature.

The overnight dexamethasone suppression test is an effective screening test for endogenous Cushing's syndrome and is suitable for the study of outpatients. In this test, 1.0 mg of dexamethasone is given orally at 2300 to 2400, and the plasma cortisol is measured at 0800 the following morning. In normal subjects, the early morning surge of ACTH secretion is obliterated by this dose of dexamethasone and the 0800 plasma cortisol is generally 5 μg/100 ml or less. In patients with Cushing's syndrome, cortisol secretion is not suppressed, and the post-dexamethasone 0800 plasma cortisol concentration usually exceeds 10 μg/100 ml (Fig. 4-5). Results of this test have been found to be abnormal in 97% of patients with recognized Cushing's syndrome. False positive results do occur, especially if the test is performed incorrectly. The tim-

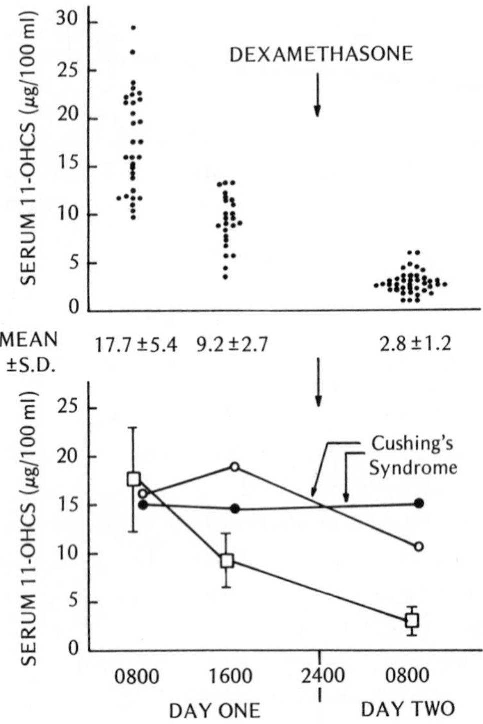

FIG. 4-5. Diurnal variation and overnight dexamethasone suppression tests in 39 subjects without adrenocortical disease (individual values upper graph, mean values lower graph). The values from two patients with Cushing's syndrome are superimposed in the lower graph. (From PE Cryer, J Sode, R Hines et al: *Med Ann DC* 39:570, 1970.)

ing of dexamethasone administration (2300-2400) is critical; the drug should not be given early in the evening. It must be given orally, since inadequate suppression may result if it is administered by intravenous injection. Patients with accelerated metabolic clearance of cortisol (and dexamethasone) may not suppress normally after the standard 1.0 mg dose. Included are patients with thyrotoxicosis and patients chronically treated with drugs that induce hepatic enzymes (barbiturates, diphenylhydantoin, phenylbutazone, etc.). Some clinicians advocate routine administration of a hypnotic on the night of the test, since an anxious patient who is unable to sleep may not suppress normally (stress can cause ACTH release even in the presence of elevated levels of circulating glucocorticoids). The overnight dexamethasone suppression test generally is valid in patients with elevated plasma CBG levels (e.g., from estrogen ingestion in the form of oral contraceptives), although nonsuppressed plasma cortisol concentrations will be somewhat elevated in these patients, mean suppressed levels are somewhat higher and false positive tests somewhat more frequent.

Even when the overnight dexamethasone suppression test is performed correctly, false positives do occur, particularly in obese patients. Some endocrinologists administer a larger dose of dexamethasone to obese patients, but the author is not aware of careful studies documenting that this larger dose does not increase the incidence of false negative tests. Since the overnight dexamethasone suppression test is a *screening* test, false negatives must be scrupulously avoided, even at the expense of some false positives. Therefore, the 1.0 mg test should be used. Patients who fail to show suppression should be further evaluated, preferably by the measurement of urinary cortisol as described below.

Base-line urinary 17-OHCS (in milligrams per 24 hours) are normal in at least 15% of patients with Cushing's syndrome and borderline in many more. Some of this overlap is due to the normal relationship between cortisol secretion and lean body mass, which allows a broad normal range. Somewhat better discrimination between normal subjects and patients with Cushing's syndrome can be achieved if the urinary 17-OHCS in a complete 24-hour collection are expressed in milligrams per gram of creatinine. Normal urinary 17-OHCS are usually less than 7 mg/gm creatinine, whereas patients with Cushing's syndrome usually excrete more than 10 mg/gm creatinine. It should be emphasized that, even with a "standardized" test like the urinary 17-OHCS, normal values vary from laboratory to laboratory.

In contrast to the urinary 17-OHCS, the 24-hour urinary cortisol (urinary "free" cortisol) excretion is *distinctly* elevated in over 90% of patients with Cushing's syndrome. The urinary cortisol directly reflects the free (unbound) cortisol concentration in plasma, which increases disproportionately when total plasma cortisol levels exceed the level of CBG saturation (usually about 20 μg/100 ml). When competitive binding methods are used, normal, non-stressed, and non-pregnant individuals excrete less than 100 μg of cortisol in the urine daily. Persistently normal urinary cortisol excretion excludes the diagnosis of endogenous Cushing's syndrome (low levels are seen in exogenous Cushing's syndrome). When base-line cortisol excretion is elevated, one should proceed to the formal dexamethasone suppression test for confirmation of the presence of Cushing's syndrome and possible clarification of its mechanism. This test is performed as follows:

Day 1. Base-line 24-hour urinary cortisol (or 17-OHCS).*
Day 2. Base-line 24-hour urinary cortisol (or 17-OHCS).
Day 3. Low-dose (0.5 mg Q6H) dexamethasone with 24-hour urinary cortisol (or 17-OHCS).
Day 4. Low-dose (0.5 mg Q6H) dexamethasone with 24-hour urinary cortisol (or 17-OHCS). Failure of the cortisols (or 17-OHCS) to suppress to normal is indicative of Cushing's syndrome.

* As discussed earlier, the creatinine content should be measured in all 24-hour urine collections. It is customary, although not critical, to also measure the 17-KS in base-line urine samples, since markedly elevated 17-KS occur in some patients with functioning adrenocortical carcinomas. The urine sample for cortisol should not contain preservative.

Day 5. High-dose (2.0 mg Q6H) dexamethasone with 24-hour urinary cortisol (or 17-OHCS).

Day 6. High-dose (2.0 mg Q6H) dexamethasone with 24-hour urinary cortisol (or 17-OHCS). Failure of the cortisol (or 17-OHCS) to suppress suggests the presence of a functioning adrenocortical tumor (or tumors) or the ectopic ACTH syndrome. Suppression (in the presence of failure to suppress during low-dose dexamethasone) is indicative of Cushing's disease.

Although normal values should be established for each laboratory, data from a rather extensive experience with Cushing's syndrome provide a frame of reference. Eddy and co-workers compared the 24-hour urinary cortisol excretion (by competitive binding analysis) in 24 patients with Cushing's syndrome with that of 15 controls with "Cushingoid obesity." Base-line cortisol excretion ranged from 138 to 1462 μg/24 hours in the patients with Cushing's syndrome and from 11 to 102 μg/24 hours in the controls. On the second day of low-dose dexamethasone administration, cortisol excretion fell to less than 20 μg/24 hours in the controls and ranged from 127 to 1613 μg/24 hours in the patients with Cushing's syndrome. On the second day of high-dose dexamethasone administration, cortisol excretion fell to less than 50% of the base-line values in eight of ten patients with Cushing's disease, none of ten patients with functioning adrenocortical tumors, and none of ten patients with ectopic ACTH secretion.

A urinary 17-OHCS value of less than 4.0 mg/24 hours (or 2.5 mg/gm creatinine) on the second day of low-dose dexamethasone administration is considered normal by many authorities. But as noted, normal 17-OHCS values vary somewhat from laboratory to laboratory.

Rarely, the diagnosis of Cushing's disease (Cushing's syndrome due to excessive pituitary ACTH secretion) can be made, on the basis of convincing clinical evidence and persistently elevated base-line urinary cortisol excretion, despite normal suppression during the administration of a pharmacologic dose (0.5 mg every

6 hours–the standard "low dose") of dexamethasone. This diagnosis should be made with great caution, however, since normal subjects may have urinary cortisol values that approach 300 μg/24 hours when under severe psychic or physical stress. If the clinical circumstances are not pressing, this diagnosis should be made only after serial re-evaluation of the patient over several months.

Measurement of plasma ACTH can facilitate etiologic diagnosis in patients with Cushing's syndrome, particularly when the plasma ACTH is markedly elevated (ectopic ACTH syndrome). Although groups of patients with Cushing's disease have been found to have elevated plasma ACTH levels, and patients with Cushing's syndrome due to adrenocortical tumors (or exogenous glucocorticoid administration) have suppressed plasma ACTH levels, the values for individual patients in these groups may not be readily distinguishable from normal. In addition, it is at least theoretically possible that some patients with the ectopic ACTH syndrome will be found to secrete a biologically active, non-immunoreactive ACTH-like molecule.

Once Cushing's syndrome is suspected, diagnosis of the ectopic ACTH syndrome is usually not difficult. The primary tumor (commonly in the lung) is often overt, and evidence of metastases is the rule. Clinical features favoring this diagnosis include weight loss and disproportionate weakness, hyperpigmentation, edema, hypokalemia, and markedly elevated base-line plasma and urinary steroid values. Occasionally, clinically apparent Cushing's syndrome precedes the clinically apparent tumor, and a failure to demonstrate high-dose dexamethasone suppression suggests the presence of an adrenocortical tumor, with the correct diagnosis being made only when bilateral adrenocortical hyperplasia is found at laparotomy. Since, as mentioned above, the distinction between Cushing's syndrome due to an adrenocortical tumor and that due to ectopic ACTH secretion can usually be made preoperatively by measurement of the plasma ACTH level, this error is avoidable. Although tumors of the lung, pancreas, and thymus are the most frequent sources, ectopic ACTH secretion from a wide variety of tumors has been recognized. The production of Cushing's syndrome by bronchial carcinoids deserves special comment, since, in sharp contrast to the typical ectopic ACTH syndrome, suppression of cortisol excretion during high-dose dexamethasone administration has been observed in roughly one-half the patients.

Ancillary tests in patients with Cushing's syndrome include estimates of bone density (bone densitometry, X-rays of the spine) and a glucose tolerance test, which indicate the intensity of the disease and provide base-line data. Skull films are important in patients with Cushing's disease, since the finding of an enlarged sella turcica may determine the therapeutic approach.

In summary, when Cushing's syndrome is suspected (and when there has been no ingestion of exogenous glucocorticoids) an overnight dexamethasone suppression test should be performed. If the post-dexamethasone 0800 plasma cortisol is 5 μg/100 ml or less, the diagnosis is rejected. If this value is greater than 5 μg/100 ml, measurements of 24-hour urinary cortisol excretion should be obtained. If cortisol excretion is persistently normal, the diagnosis is rejected. If cortisol excretion is elevated, a formal dexamethasone suppression test is performed. Failure of suppression of cortisol excretion during the administration of low-dose dexamethasone confirms the diagnosis of Cushing's syndrome. Failure of suppression of cortisol excretion during high-dose dexamethasone administration suggests that the Cushing's syndrome is due to ectopic ACTH secretion or an adrenal tumor (or tumors). The later disorders can be distinguished by measuring the plasma ACTH concentration. Suppression of cortisol excretion during high-dose dexamethasone administration (after absence of suppression during low-dose dexamethasone administration) is typical of Cushing's disease.

Adrenocortical insufficiency may be due to primary adrenocortical disease (Addison's disease) or deficient pituitary ACTH secretion, which may occur as an isolated deficiency or as one component of a deficiency of multiple pituitary hormones (hypopituitarism). A not uncommon form of isolated ACTH deficiency is that following termination of chronic glucocorticoid therapy, originally administered for non-endocrine disease. The differential diagnosis of hypopituitarism is discussed in Chapter 2. Primary adrenocortical insufficiency is most often idiopathic (perhaps autoimmune) or due to infectious destruction of the glands, particularly as a result of tuberculosis or histoplasmosis. Other causes include adrenal hemorrhage (due to anticoagulant therapy, sepsis, or trauma), amyloidosis, metastatic disease, and of course, adrenalectomy.

Patients with primary adrenocortical insufficiency (Addison's disease) are deficient in both glucocorticoid and mineralocorticoid secretion. ACTH-deficient patients have inadequate glucocorticoid secretion; their mineralocorticoid secretion is usually adequate. Loss of axillary and pubic hair in women with adrenocortical insufficiency reflects a loss of adrenal androgen secretion.

In some instances, *primary adrenocortical insufficiency* is rather easily diagnosed—the patient has compatible symptoms and signs, definite hyperpigmentation, hyperkalemia, and an 0800 plasma cortisol of less than 3 μg/100 ml. The administration of ACTH (synthetic α1-24 ACTH, cosyntropin, 250 μg intramuscularly or intravenously with plasma cortisols measured at zero time and at 60 and 120 minutes after injection) demonstrates a failure of the cortisol response and is confirmatory (Fig. 4-6). If the patient is suspected to be in Addisonian crisis, this ACTH test (ACTH given intravenously) can be performed simultaneously with therapy with a potent synthetic glucocorticoid, such as dexamethasone (which will not alter the subsequent plasma cortisol determinations), and appropriate sodium-containing fluids.

In other instances, the clinical picture is not as clear cut, the 0800 plasma cortisol overlaps the normal range, and the ACTH test becomes more critical. In patients who do not have Addison's disease, the plasma cortisol concentration will rise by at least 10 μg/100 ml after ACTH, whereas no change occurs in patients who have Addison's disease.

Mineralocorticoid deficiency in Addison's disease is reflected in clinical evidence of volume contraction (often with hypona-

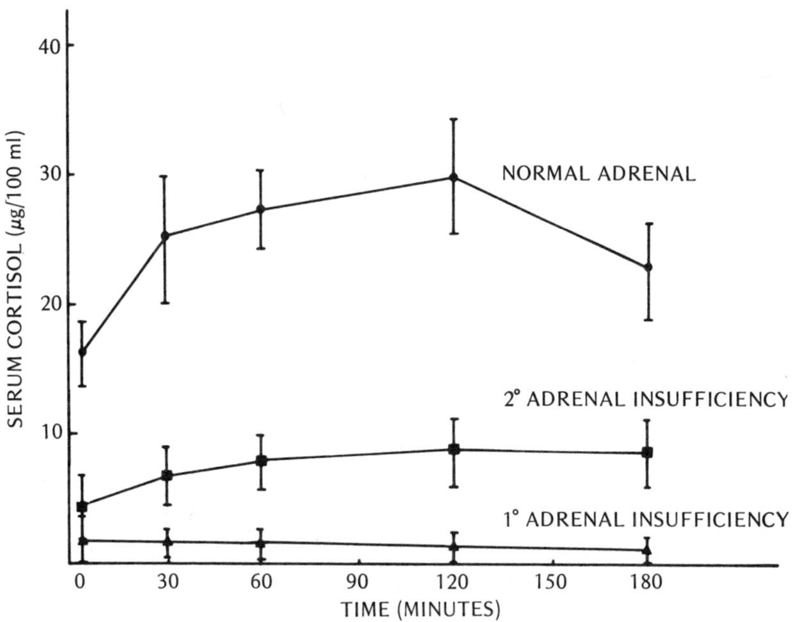

FIG. 4-6. Serum cortisol response to synthetic adrenocorticotropin (cosyntropin) in normal subjects and in patients with primary and secondary adrenocortical insufficiency. (From Speckart PF, Nicoloff JT, Bethune JE: *Arch Int Med* 128:761, 1971.)

tremia) and in the presence of hyperkalemia. Aldosterone levels are not routinely measured but are low in patients with Addison's disease.

In considering ancillary studies, one should keep the conditions sometimes associated with Addison's disease (including hypothyroidism, hypoparathyroidism, hypogonadism, diabetes, and pernicious anemia) in mind.

Inadequate ACTH secretion from the pituitary results in *secondary adrenocortical insufficiency* (which may result from either pituitary or hypothalamic disease) manifested by the clinical effects of glucocorticoid deficit. In patients with an established deficiency of multiple pituitary hormones, symptoms and signs compatible with glucocorticoid deficiency, and an 0800 plasma cortisol level of less than 3 μg/100 ml, the diagnosis of secondary adrenocortical insufficiency is often presumed. Tests of ACTH reserve, specifically the metyrapone test, are unnecessary (since the plasma cortisol is already low) and may precipitate acute adrenocortical insufficiency. The diagnosis of secondary adrenocortical insufficiency is not conclusively established, however, until the capacity of the adrenal cortex to respond to exogenous ACTH is demonstrated. Some patients have a definite (but subnormal) increase in the plasma cortisol 60 and 120 minutes after cosyntropin, and this distinguishes them from patients with primary adrenocortical insufficiency (Fig. 4-6). Other patients, particularly those with long-standing ACTH lack (including patients treated for several years with exogenous glucocorticoids), may not have a demonstrable response to this short test and will require prolonged ACTH infusion. The continuous infusion of cosyntropin (250 μg/12 hours) for 48 hours, with measurement of urinary and/or plasma cortisols, can be used here.

In patients with suspected secondary adrenocortical insufficiency, but an 0800 plasma cortisol value of greater than 3 μg/100 ml, a test of ACTH reserve, such as the metyrapone test, is indicated. Metyrapone (Metopirone, SU-4885) is a competitive inhibitor of C_{11} hydroxylation and thus inhibits the conversion of 11-deoxycortisol to cortisol. In normal subjects, the resulting decrease in plasma cortisol triggers an increase in ACTH secretion, with a consequent increase in adrenal steroid synthesis and release of the intermediate proximal to the enzymatic block (11-deoxycortisol) into the blood and urine. 11-Deoxycortisol can be measured indirectly as a 17-OHCS in the urine or more specifically in urine or plasma.

The metyrapone test has been simplified by the development of methods for selective extraction and measurement of 11-deoxycortisol (compound S) in plasma. This can be performed by extraction of 11-deoxycortisol with benzene (cortisol is not extracted in this solvent) and by performance of a competitive binding analysis with 11-deoxycortisol standards. Following the administration of metyrapone (750 mg orally every 4 hours for six doses starting at 0800), the 0800 plasma 11-deoxycortisol level rises from base-line levels of less than 3 μg/100 ml to well over 10 μg/100 ml in normal subjects, whereas the post-metyrapone value is less than 8 μg/100 ml in patients with diminished ACTH reserve (secondary adrenocortical insufficiency) as illustrated in Fig. 4-7.

Failure of the post-metyrapone plasma 11-deoxycortisol to rise does not conclusively establish diminished ACTH reserve, since the same result occurs in patients in whom inadequate blockade of C_{11} hydroxylation is produced. This can occur, for example, if only one dose of metyrapone is omitted (most often the 0400 dose). Specific measurement of cortisol in the pre- and post-metyrapone plasma samples (*after* 11-deoxycortisol extraction) documenting a fall in plasma cortisol after metyrapone adminis-

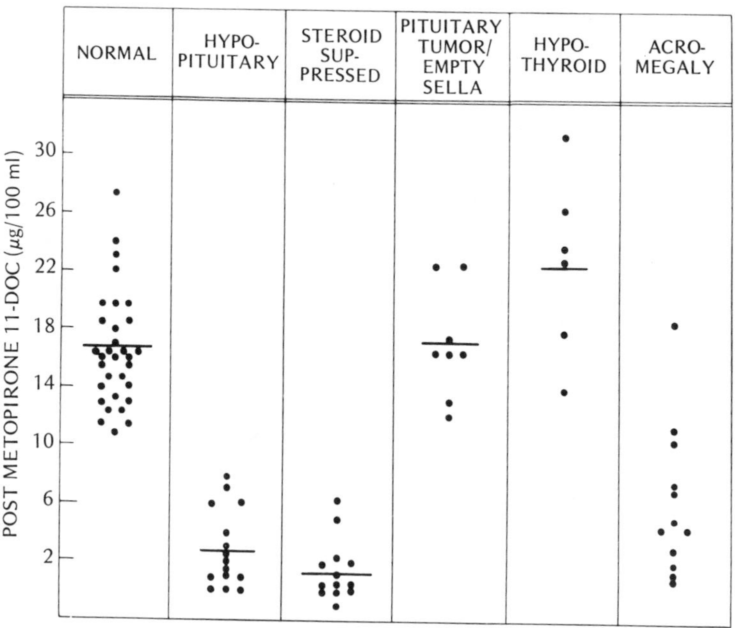

FIG. 4-7. Effects of oral metyrapone (Metopirone) on the 0800 serum 11-deoxycortisol (compound S) levels. (From Spark RF: *Ann Int Med* 75:717, 1971.)

tration confirms the production of C_{11} blockade and makes a failure of the post-metyrapone 11-deoxycortisol level to rise virtually diagnostic of diminished ACTH reserve. Since patients with primary adrenocortical insufficiency would not be expected to respond to metyrapone, the demonstration of adrenocortical responsiveness to exogenous ACTH is required to conclusively establish the diagnosis of secondary adrenocortical insufficiency in a metapyrone non-responder. This step, however, can reasonably be omitted when the clinical picture is clearly that of secondary, rather than primary, disease.

Although the author continues to use the multiple-dose metyrapone test described above, others have found a single dose-test (30 mg/kg body weight at 2400) equally effective.

The metyrapone test is a sensitive test designed to detect partial, and sometimes subtle, deficits in the capacity to secrete ACTH in response to decreased negative feedback. As mentioned earlier, it is not indicated when the diagnosis of secondary adrenocortical insufficiency is apparent from the clinical picture and base-line cortisol measurements. Although it can be concluded that the hypothalamic-pituitary-adrenocortical axis is intact in a patient who has a normal 11-deoxycortisol response to metyrapone, a subnormal response to metyrapone does not necessarily imply that the patient will not have an ACTH and cortisol response to stress. It could be reasoned that, in a patient who is clinically well despite evidence of diminished ACTH secretory reserve, a more clinically relevant question is whether the patient can respond to stress. Measurement of the plasma cortisol response to insulin-induced hypoglycemia (0.1 units/kg body weight of regular insulin with measurement of plasma glucose and cortisol at 0, 20, 40, 60, 90, and 120 minutes) can be used to answer this question. It should be recalled that this test, which can be unpleasant for the patient, requires constant physician attendance so that manifestations of neuroglycopenia can be promptly treated with intravenous glucose.

The increasing availability of improved radioimmunoassays of plasma ACTH can be expected to greatly simplify the diagnosis of adrenocortical insufficiency. Patients with primary adrenocortical insufficiency have low morning plasma cortisol levels with elevated plasma ACTH levels. Patients with fully developed secondary adrenocortical insufficiency have low morning plasma cortisol and ACTH levels.

In summary, when adrenocortical insufficiency is suspected, an 0800 plasma cortisol should be drawn. A clearly normal value excludes the diagnosis for practical purposes, whereas an 0800 value reproducibly less than 3 μg/100 ml (in the absence of exogenous glucocorticoid ingestion) is virtually diagnostic. Patients with intermediate values may have partial adrenocortical insufficiency. When primary adrenocortical insufficiency (Addison's disease) is suspected clinically, the plasma cortisol should be measured 60 and 120 minutes after cosyntropin injection. The absence of a plasma cortisol response confirms the diagnosis. When secondary adrenocortical insufficiency is suspected clinically, and the 0800 plasma cortisol is in the intermediate range, the plasma 11-deoxycortisol level should be measured before and after metyrapone administration. Failure of the plasma 11-deoxycortisol to rise after metyrapone suggests the diagnosis, although a firm confirmation requires the demonstration that an effective blockade was indeed produced by the metyrapone and that the adrenal cortex is capable of responding to exogenous ACTH.

Secondary adrenocortical insufficiency can result from disease of the anterior pituitary or the hypothalamus. It is often impossible to distinguish between these possibilities with currently available functional testing, but under certain circumstances, it can be inferred that the disorder lies at the hypothalamic level. For example, a patient with secondary adrenocortical insufficiency and elevated serum prolactin levels (not explicable on the basis of drug ingestion or pituitary tumor) probably has a hypothalamic disorder with impaired hypothalamic production of both prolactin inhibiting factor (PIF) and corticotropin releasing factor (CRF). Similarly, associated secondary hypothyroidism with a normal plasma TSH response to intravenous thyrotropin releasing hormone (TRH) indirectly favors hypothalamic localization of disease in a patient with secondary adrenocortical insufficiency. The distinction between pituitary and hypothalamic disorders is not as yet of practical therapeutic importance but may have etiologic implications.

ANDROGEN DISORDERS Excessive adrenocortical production of testosterone and/or testosterone precursors (androstenedione and dehydroepiandrosterone) occurs in patients with certain discrete enzymatic defects in cortisol synthesis (the adrenogenital syndromes), with a poorly defined syndrome of adrenocortical androgen overproduction but no recognized enzymatic defects (the postpubertal or adult adrenogenital syndrome), or with virilizing adrenocortical tumors.

Discrete enzymatic defects in cortisol synthesis characterize the *adrenogenital syndromes.* Complete absence of enzymatic activity produces lethal cortisol deficiency. Partial enzymatic defects, however, may be compensated by marked increases in ACTH secretion resulting in adequate cortisol production at the expense of gross overproduction of the steroid intermediates proximal to the enzymatic block and conversion of these intermediates to metabolically active steroid hormones. These steroid abnormalities are corrected by the administration of glucocorticoids in replacement doses. The enzymatic steps in adrenocortical biosynthesis are illustrated in Fig. 4-2.

Partial deficiencies of 21-hydroxylase or of 11-hydroxylase produce virilizing adrenogenital syndromes (classical congenital adrenal hyperplasia) due to unimpeded overproduction of adrenocortical androgens. Characteristically, these defects result in female pseudohermaphroditism (labial fusion and clitoral enlargement) in the newborn genetic female or premature virilization (often distinguished from true premature puberty by the absence of testicular enlargement) in the young male. There is a broad spectrum of clinical expression, presumably reflecting the degree of enzyme deficiency, and patients with little evidence of abnormal virilization, but typical biochemical patterns, have occasionally been detected in adult life.

Biochemically, patients with virilizing adrenogenital syndromes have distinctly elevated serum testosterone levels and urinary 17-KS. Patients with a 21-hydroxylase deficiency have normal or low urinary 17-OHCS (and cortisol) but markedly elevated levels of urinary pregnanetriol, the reduced metabolite of 17α-hydroxy-progesterone, and of plasma 17α-hydroxyprogesterone, which is the intermediate proximal to the defective enzymatic step. Patients with more severe 21-hydroxylase defects exhibit major urinary sodium loss, perhaps as a result of inadequate aldosterone secretion, competition by accumulated progesterone with mineralocorticoids for receptor sites at the distal renal tubules, or both.

Patients with a 11-hydroxylase deficiency have elevated urinary 17-OHCS (11-deoxycortisol possesses the 17,21-dihydroxy-20-keto group and is thus measured as a Porter-Silber chromogen) and elevated plasma and urine 11-deoxycortisol (compound S) levels. In contrast to the 21-hydroxylase deficiency, the 11-hydroxylase defect may result in excessive mineralocorticoid (11-deoxycorticosterone) production with resulting sodium retention and hypertension.

Other steroid biosynthetic enzyme deficiencies do not result in major androgen overproduction. Indeed, since the enzymatic steps involved are common to both the adrenal cortex and the gonad, deficient sex steroid production may result. For example, 17-hydroxylase deficiency results in overproduction of 11-deoxy-corticosterone (with resulting hypertension, hypokalemia, and suppressed plasma renin activity) plus diminished testosterone production in the male (male pseudohermaphroditism or defective pubertal virilization) and diminished estrogen production in the female (defective pubertal feminization). Other rare congenital enzymatic defects in steroid biosynthesis include 20,22 desmolase deficiency (diminished conversion of cholesterol to pregnenolone leading to decreased production of all adrenocortical and gonadal steroids), 3β-hydroxysteroid dehydrogenase deficiency (leading to decreased production of the major adrenocortical and gonadal steroids although DHA is overproduced), and 18-hydroxylase deficiency (leading to decreased aldosterone production).

Androgen overproduction of postpubertal onset, even when it can be demonstrated biochemically, is not a clinically recognizable problem in the adult male. But in the adult female, subtle androgen overproduction may be clinically apparent at a time when sophisticated studies of testosterone kinetics are required to confirm the abnormality biochemically.

Women with androgen-producing tumors of the adrenal cortex or ovary most often present with frank virilization, including clitoral enlargement, increased muscle mass, deepened voice, and temporal balding. But, hormone production by neoplastic tissue may be inefficient, and it is the first obligation of the physician who sees a patient with evidence of androgen overproduction—even when limited to hirsutism, acne, and irregular menses—to exclude an adrenocortical or ovarian tumor.

Virilizing adrenocortical tumors are usually excluded biochemically, since androgen-producing tumors of the adrenal cortex usually secrete milligram quantities of DHA and its metabolites, resulting in elevated urinary 17-KS. Normal urinary 17-KS, or suppression of elevated urinary 17-KS to less than 50% of base line with dexamethasone (i.e., 1.0 mg upon retiring for 7 to 10 days), excludes androgen-producing adrenocortical tumor for practical purposes.*

Virilizing ovarian tumors, in contrast, are excluded on an anatomic basis. The absence of an adnexal mass on careful pelvic examination is usually sufficient, although in some obese patients, pneumogynegrams, or laparoscopy, is required. Virilizing ovarian tumors are not invariably palpable, and the preceding procedures may be indicated when the clinical suspicion of ovarian tumor is high (i.e., rapidly progressive or intense virilization or the occurrence of androgen excess in young girls or middle-aged or older women associated with relatively normal 17-KS excretion).

The vast majority of women with hirsutism, acne, and irregular

* A few patients with normal urinary 17-KS and a testosterone-producing tumor that was adrenocortical in location (but gonadal in behavior, i.e., responsive to injected chorionic gonadotropins) have been reported recently.

menses without other clinical evidence of androgen overproduction do not have adrenocortical or ovarian tumors, nor do they have Cushing's syndrome or any of the recognized enzymatic defects in cortisol synthesis.* Nonetheless, testosterone production rates (calculated from the product of the measured metabolic clearance rate of infused labeled testosterone and the serum testosterone concentration) are elevated in these patients, confirming the presence of androgen overproduction.

Endocrinologists have traditionally attempted to categorize such patients on the basis of the origin–adrenocortical or ovarian –of androgen overproduction. Patients with a presumed adrenocortical androgen source (usually based upon dexamethasone suppressibility of elevated urinary 17-KS, serum testosterone, or both) were felt to have the adult (or postpubertal) adrenogenital syndrome; patients with a presumed ovarian androgen source (usually based upon ovarian enlargement, abnormal histology, and/or estrogen suppressibility or gonadotropin stimulatability of serum testosterone) were felt to have the polycystic (sclerocystic) ovary syndrome (Stein-Leventhal syndrome) or a variant thereof. But ovarian and adrenal vein catheterization studies of hirsute women with normal or slightly elevated urinary 17-KS have led to several relevant observations: First, the ovary is a common origin of androgen overproduction. Second, combined adrenocortical and ovarian androgen overproduction is not uncommon. Third, the results of suppression tests correlate poorly with the more direct catheterization findings in terms of the source of androgen overproduction. Thus, although the designation "adult adrenogenital syndrome" may be appropriate in patients with distinctly elevated urinary 17-KS (greater than 20 mg/24 hours), which suppress normally, the remaining large group of patients should be considered to have *idiopathic androgen overproduction* in the absence of definitive catheterization data.

In summary, postpubertal women with evidence of androgen

* Evidence that partial 21- or 11-hydroxylase deficiencies can be recognized in at least some of these patients has been reported (Newmark SR, Dluhy RG, Williams GH et al.: *Clin Res* 23:240A, 1975).

overproduction should have their urinary 17-KS and serum testosterone levels measured, in addition to a physical examination that includes a careful pelvic examination. If the urinary 17-KS are elevated, dexamethasone suppressibility must be demonstrated. The measurement of urinary pregnanetriol and plasma 11-deoxycortisol adds to the expense and has a very low diagnostic yield. If Cushing's syndrome is suggested clinically, an overnight dexamethasone suppression test is indicated.

The serum testosterone concentration is elevated in the majority of women with androgen overproduction and provides biochemical confirmation of the diagnosis as well as an objective means of evaluating therapy. Unfortunately, the base-line total serum testosterone concentration is not elevated in all patients (even when elevated testosterone production rates can be demonstrated by the clearance technique). This apparent paradox may be due to an increase in the fraction of circulating testosterone not bound to testosterone binding globulin (with a corresponding decrease in bound testosterone), since it is the unbound fraction that is available to the tissues to produce androgenic effects. Thus, it is reasonable to measure the free, as well as the total, serum testosterone concentration in women with evidence of androgen excess.

It should be recalled that the serum testosterone concentration is not a feedback-regulated variable in women; its serum concentration merely passively reflects the balance between testosterone influx into and efflux from the circulation. Thus, factors that increase testosterone clearance or decrease testosterone binding or both (androgen excess, glucocorticoids, progestins, hypothyroidism) would be expected to lower the serum level of testosterone, whereas factors that decrease testosterone clearance or increase testosterone binding or both (estrogen administration or overproduction, especially during pregnancy, cirrhosis, hyperthyroidism) would be expected to raise its serum level.

Deficient adrenocortical androgen secretion is not a clinically recognizable problem in men with normal testes. In contrast, women with deficient adrenocortical androgen production (as in adrenocortical insufficiency) may exhibit diminished growth of pubic and axillary hair.

MINERALOCORTICOID DISORDERS Aldosterone, the principal mineralocorticoid, is produced by the zona glomerulosa of the adrenal cortex. Its secretion is regulated primarily by the renin-angiotensin system (in response to changes in effective blood volume), although the serum potassium concentration exerts a direct influence on aldosterone secretion. ACTH plays a relatively minor role in the regulation of aldosterone secretion, but the production of other mineralocorticoids, notably 11-deoxycorticosterone (DOC), from the fasciculata and reticularis of the adrenal cortex is a direct reflection of the plasma ACTH level. The major factors regulating aldosterone secretion are illustrated diagrammatically in Fig. 4-8.

Chronic excessive mineralocorticoid secretion results in sodium retention and hypertension, plus renal potassium wasting that often leads to hypokalemia and alkalosis. Excessive 11-deoxycorticosterone secretion occurs in some cases of ACTH-dependent Cushing's syndrome (Cushing's disease and the ectopic ACTH syndrome), in some patients with adrenocortical tumors, and in those with the C11-hydroxylase and C17-hydroxylase deficiency syndromes (where it is associated with virilization and defective sexual development, respectively, and is eradicated by suppressive doses of glucocorticoids). Hypertension due to 11-deoxycorticosterone overproduction occurs less frequently than that due to aldosterone overproduction, primary aldosteronism.

Primary aldosteronism is a syndrome characterized by hypertension with potassium wasting, increased aldosterone secretion, and suppressed renin secretion. It can be caused by an aldosterone-producing adenoma* (APA) or by hyperplasia of the adrenal cortex. Biglieri has further subdivided primary aldosteronism due to adrenocortical hyperplasia into three categories: (a) idiopathic hyperaldosteronism (IHA), (b) indeterminant hyperaldoste-

* Rarely, primary aldosteronism has been found to be caused by an adrenocortical carcinoma or a gonadal tumor.

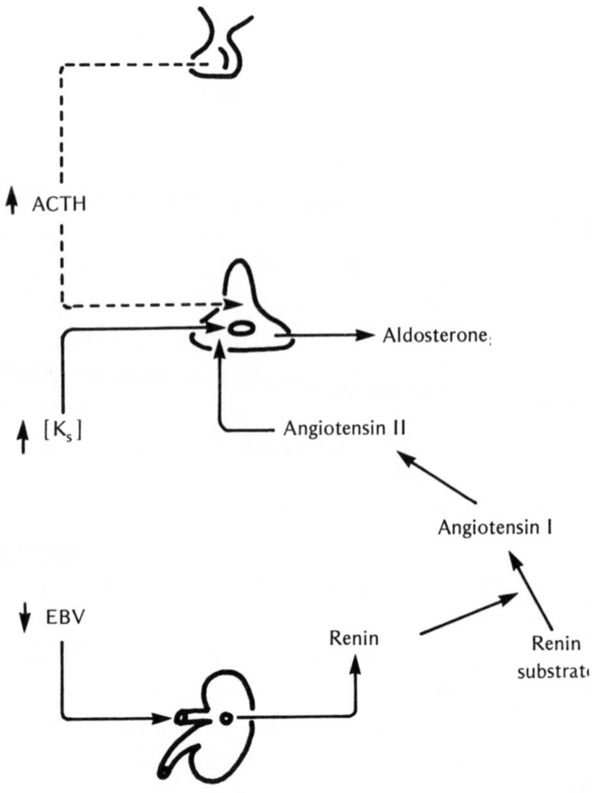

FIG. 4-8. Major factors regulating aldosterone secretion; EBV, effective blood volume.

ronism (InHA) characterized by elevated base-line aldosterone levels, which suppress normally during sodium loading, and (c) the rare glucocorticoid-remedial hyperaldosteronism (GRHA) in which the hypertension and biochemical abnormalities are corrected by the administration of suppressive doses of a glucocorticoid, such as dexamethasone. Once the diagnosis of primary aldosteronism is established, however, the fundamental clinical distinction is between APA—a potentially surgically curable lesion—and hyperplasia, which is not amenable to surgical therapy.

Although its true prevalence is not known, primary aldosteronism is not a common cause of hypertension. The major clinical problem, then, is how to select patients with primary aldosteronism from the large population of patients with hypertension of other etiologies. Unexplained hypokalemia in the hypertensive patient is the calling card of primary aldosteronism, although the disease has been recognized in patients without hypokalemia. The latter patients become hypokalemic, however, during sodium loading. A urinary potassium of less than 30 mEq/24 hours in a hypokalemic patient strongly suggests that the hypokalemia is not due to an excessive mineralocorticoid effect at the renal tubule. In contrast, a urinary potassium of greater than 40 mEq/24 hours in a hypokalemic hypertensive patient not on therapy is an absolute indication for definitive diagnostic testing—including aldosterone and renin activity determinations—for primary aldosteronism. It should be emphasized that the occurrence of thiazide-induced hypokalemia is not a reliable clue to the presence of underlying primary aldosteronism. The serum potassium determination should be repeated several weeks following termination of thiazide therapy. If hypokalemia persists, the urinary potassium should be measured (after potassium chloride replacement therapy has been terminated), as described above.

Given the presence of hypertension and potassium wasting, and the absence of the clinical features of the disorders associated with 11-deoxycorticosterone overproduction listed earlier, the definitive diagnostic evaluation should be designed to establish the presence of primary aldosteronism and to determine whether it is due to an APA or to hyperplasia. Initially, this should include (a) measurement, with the patient ingesting a sodium sufficient diet (i.e., $>$ 120 mEq per day), of the overnight supine plasma aldosterone concentration (or 24-hour urinary aldosterone excretion), (b) measurement of the plasma (or urinary) aldosterone response to sodium loading, (c) measurement of the plasma aldosterone response to upright activity, and (d) measurement of the plasma renin activity (PRA) response to sodium depletion and upright activity.

In general, patients with APA have more striking biochemical abnormalities—lower serum potassium levels, a lower PRA, often with no measurable response to provocative maneuvers, and higher aldosterone levels—than patients with hyperplasia. For example, an overnight supine plasma aldosterone concentration, in a sodium sufficient patient, over 20 ng/dl favors APA, whereas patients with hyperplasia more often have aldosterone levels, although elevated, under 20 ng/dl. Patients with APA and patients with IHA fail to exhibit suppression of aldosterone levels during sodium loading, whereas elevated but suppressible aldosterone levels define InHA. The classic approach to sodium loading involves measurement of aldosterone levels before and after 3 days of a high sodium diet coupled with the administration of deoxycorticosterone acetate, 10 mg intramuscularly every 12 hours (the DOCA suppression test). But this test is time consuming and hypertension and hypokalemia may worsen during its performance. Streeten and his colleagues have found that a supine plasma aldosterone concentration greater than 8 ng/dl after 2 liters of intravenous saline over 4 hours, especially when coupled with spontaneous hypokalemia and suppressed PRA, accurately predicted failure to respond to the DOCA suppression test. As mentioned earlier, plasma aldosterone concentrations normally rise during upright activity. Patients with primary aldosteronism as a result of hyperplasia also exhibit this pattern. In contrast, patients with APA commonly, but not invariably, exhibit a decrease (or no change) in plasma aldosterone during upright activity.

The author's approach to the formal evaluation of the patient with hypertension, spontaneous hypokalemia, and urinary potassium wasting (in the absence of disorders associated with 11-deoxycorticosterone overproduction) is as follows:

Day 1. Measurement of the overnight supine morning plasma aldosterone level and the supine plasma aldosterone level after 2 liters of intravenous saline over 4 hours.

Day 2. Measurement of the overnight supine morning plasma aldosterone level and the plasma aldosterone level after 4 hours of upright activity. After the second sample, furosemide 80 mg is given orally and dietary sodium is restricted (to less than 20 mEq/day) through the Day 3 study.

Day 3. Measurement of PRA after 4 hours of upright activity.

The findings of elevated supine plasma aldosterone concentrations and suppressed PRA define the syndrome of primary aldosteronism and failure of the plasma aldosterone level to suppress during saline infusion excludes InHA. Marked biochemical abnormalities and a decrease in plasma aldosterone during upright activity favor APA over IHA.

Given biochemical findings suggesting APA, attempts to anatomically lateralize the lesion are in order. Because of their noninvasive nature, computed tomographic (CT) scans of the adrenals are an appropriate first step, although they are of value only if positive, since adenomas may be small. Some investigators have found iodocholesterol scans to be of value in localizing an APA, although others have been reluctant to utilize this technique because of the relatively large radiation dose required. If technically successful, bilateral adrenal vein catheterization with samples for plasma aldosterone (as well as an adrenal vein marker, such as cortisol or epinephrine) can provide excellent, albeit indirect, evidence of the presence of an APA (steep adrenal vein to inferior vena cava aldosterone gradient on one side) or IHA (bilateral aldosterone gradients). It is critical, however, that samples be obtained from both adrenal veins, since appreciable gradients from the side contralateral to an APA can be seen. This is not a simple procedure; for example, the right adrenal vein, which normally drains directly into the vena cava, cannot be entered in 20%, or more, of patients. Furthermore, it is an invasive and expensive study. Nonetheless, since the alternative is exploratory laparotomy without lateralizing evidence—with the possibility that the surgeon will find bilateral hyperplasia rather than an adenoma

—the author continues to recommend venous catheterization when noninvasive attempts at lateralization have failed.

It should be emphasized that the finding of suppressed PRA alone is not indicative of primary aldosteronism, since this finding is present in 20% or more of patients with essential hypertension and normal or low aldosterone excretion, socalled *low-renin hypertension.* Some of these patients have been found to excrete excessive quantities of other mineralocorticoids (e.g., 18-hydroxy-11-deoxycorticosterone). Whether all patients with low renin hypertension have hypersecretion of mineralocorticoid hormones remains to be established.

The role of mineralocorticoids in the pathogenesis of *renovascular hypertension* is unclear. Aldosterone excretion is normal or only slightly elevated in many of these patients. The direct pressor effect of angiotensin II may be the cause of the hypertension. Thus, aldosterone measurements are not of value in the diagnosis of renovascular hypertension. Measurement of PRA in both renal veins, with the criterion a ratio of 1.5 or greater (side with arteriographically demonstrated renal artery stenosis over uninvolved side), despite practical limitations, remains the best available diagnostic test. Volume contraction may increase the diagnostic yield of this maneuver. Similarly, the role of mineralocorticoids in the pathogenesis of the hypertension of *primary reninism* is unknown. Patients with primary reninism have inappropriately high PRA and tumors of the renal juxtaglomerular apparatus, and their hypertension is cured by surgical removal of the involved kidney. Similar patients with ectopic renin secretion (e.g., from carcinoma of the lung) have been reported.

Aldosterone deficiency is a feature of primary adrenocortical insufficiency. *Isolated hypoaldosteronism* (manifested primarily by hyperkalemia) with normal cortisol secretion has been recognized with increasing frequency. It can be due to either a primary adrenocortical defect in aldosterone production or a defect in renin secretion. The former is characterized by elevated PRA and absence of an aldosterone response to infused angiotensin II or ACTH, whereas the latter is characterized by deficient PRA and aldosterone responses to sodium depletion/upright activity. Isolated hypoaldosteronism, generally of the hyporeninemic variety, is particularly common in diabetic patients, although multiple factors, including insulin deficiency, may well play a role in the pathogenesis of diabetic hyperkalemia.

In addition, a syndrome of mineralocorticoid resistance has been recognized in a few patients with chronic renal disease but minimal azotemia.

ESTROGEN DISORDERS Estrogen overproduction does not produce overt clinical manifestations in the adult woman (aside from menstrual abnormalities) but may result in feminization of the adult man. The most common manifestation of the latter is gynecomastia, with testicular atrophy occurring less frequently. Perhaps the most clear-cut, although not the most common, form of excessive estrogen secretion is that due to a *feminizing adrenocortical tumor.* Findings of elevated urinary or serum estrogens plus anatomic evidence of an adrenal mass in a feminized man establish the preoperative diagnosis. The differential diagnosis raised by the finding of gynecomastia is discussed more fully in Chapter 5.

SUGGESTED READING

1. Liddle GW: The adrenal cortex. *In* Textbook of Endocrinology, Fifth Edition. Williams RH (ed). Saunders, Philadelphia, 1974, p 233.
2. Bongiovanni AM: Congenital adrenal hyperplasia and related conditions. *In* The Metabolic Basis of Inherited Disease, Fourth Edition. Stanbury JB, Wyngaarden JB, Fredrickson DS (eds). McGraw-Hill, New York, 1978, p 868.
3. Eddy RL, Jones AL, Gilliland PF et al: Cushing's syndrome: A prospective study of diagnostic methods. *Amer J Med* 55:621, 1973.
4. Moore TJ, Dluhy RG, Williams GH, Cain JP: Nelson's syndrome: Frequency, prognosis and effect of prior pituitary irradiation. *Ann Intern Med* 85:731, 1976.
5. Smals AGH, Kloppenborg PWC, Benraad TJ: Plasma testosterone profiles in Cushing's syndrome. *J Clin Endocrinol Metab* 45:240, 1977.

6. Hogan MJ, Schambelan M, Biglieri EG: Concurrent hypercortisolism and hypermineralocorticoidism. *Amer J Med* 62:777, 1977.
7. Biglieri EG, Lopez JM: Clinical and laboratory diagnosis of adrenocortical hypertension. *Cardiovasc Med* 1:335, 1976.
8. Horton R, Finck E. Diagnosis and localization in primary aldosteronism. *Ann Intern Med* 76:1039, 1972.
9. Conn JW, Cohen EL, Lucas CP et al: Primary reninism. *Arch Intern Med* 130:682, 1972.
10. Esler M, Zweifler A, Randall O et al: The determinants of plasma renin activity in essential hypertension. *Ann Intern Med* 88:746, 1978.
11. Kirschner MA, Bardin CW: Androgen production and metabolism in normal and virilized women. *Metabolism* 21:667, 1972.
12. Speckart PF, Nicoloff JT, Bethune JE: Screening for adrenocortical insufficiency with cosyntropin (synthetic ACTH). *Arch Intern Med* 128:761, 1971.
13. Spark RF: Simplified assessment of pituitary-adrenal reserve: Measurement of serum 11-deoxycortisol and cortisol after metyrapone. *Ann Intern Med* 75:717, 1971.
14. Broughton A: Application of adrenocorticotropin assays in a routine clinical laboratory. *Amer J Clin Path* 64:618, 1975.
15. Michelis MF, Murdaugh HV: Selective hypoaldosteronism. *Amer J Med* 59:1, 1975.
16. Meikle AW, Tyler FH: Potency and duration of action of glucocorticoids. *Amer J Med* 63:200, 1977.
17. Fauci AS: Alternate-day corticosteroid therapy. *Amer J Med* 64:729, 1978.

5

THE GONADS

The gonads have two basic functions: to produce sex steroids (principally testosterone in men and estradiol and progesterone in women) and to form gametes (spermatozoa and ova).

The enzyme systems involved in sex steroid synthesis in the testis and ovary are similar to those of the adrenal cortex minus the 21-, 11-, and 18-hydroxylase systems (Fig. 5-1). Androstenedione, the precursor of testosterone and the estrogens, can be formed from pregnenolone via either progesterone and 17α-hydroxyprogesterone or 17α-hydroxypregnenolone and dehydroepiandrosterone (DHA). The latter pathway may be the major one. The quantity of DHA released from the gonads is, however, only 1% of that released from the adrenal cortex. Estradiol is the major estrogen secreted from the ovary. Circulating estrone is derived in large part from peripheral conversion of androstenedione of adrenocortical and gonadal origin. Testosterone is secreted directly from the testis.

Like other steroid hormones, the sex steroids are largely bound to plasma proteins in the circulation. Testosterone and estrogens are bound to a specific sex steroid binding protein (testosterone estrogen binding globulin, TeBG). Progesterone binds to corticosteroid binding globulin (CBG). It is the free (unbound) component that is available to tissues to produce the metabolic effects of the sex steroids; it also participates in the feedback control of gonadotropin secretion.

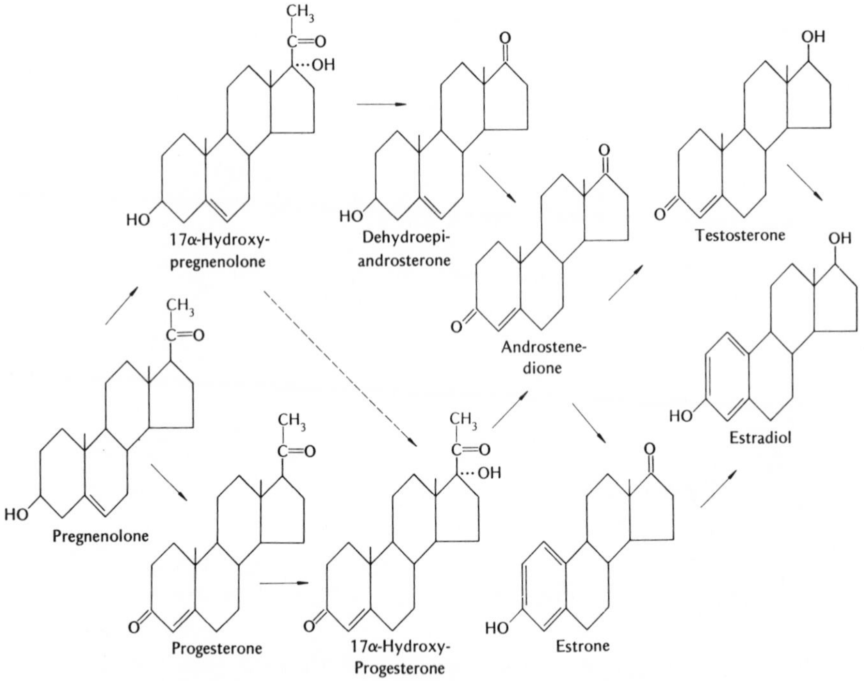

17α-Hydroxy-pregnenolone

Dehydroepi-androsterone

Androstene-dione

Testosterone

Estradiol

Pregnenolone

Progesterone

17α-Hydroxy-Progesterone

Estrone

FIG. 5-1. The sex steroids and their biosynthetic pathways.

The gonadotropins, luteinizing hormone (LH) and follicle stimulating hormone (FSH), are secreted from the anterior pituitary. As discussed in Chapter 2, the secretion of gonadotropins is modulated by one or more hypothalamic releasing hormones. Hypothalamic LH releasing hormone (LH-RH) has been synthesized and shown to release both LH and FSH in human subjects. Thus, it has been suggested that this single hypophysiotropic hormone (gonadotropin releasing hormone, Gn-RH) modulates gonadotropin secretion. But, the existence of a separate FSH releasing hormone has not been excluded.

Although the development of analytical methods based upon the competitive binding analysis principle for the measurement of gonadotropins and sex steroids has clarified the regulation of sex steroid secretion, many questions remain. In men, LH stimulates testicular Leydig cell testosterone secretion and circulating testosterone exerts a negative feedback on pituitary LH secretion, and FSH stimulates spermatogenesis, which appears to be related to the regulation of FSH secretion (i.e., azoospermic men with normal LH and testosterone levels have elevated FSH levels). The nature of the putative negative feedback relationship between spermatogenesis and FSH secretion, however, is unclear. In addition, high local testosterone concentrations within the testis are required for normal spermatogenesis.

In women, FSH promotes follicular development, and both FSH and LH are required for normal estrogen secretion. Ovulation appears to be triggered by a mid-cycle surge in LH (and FSH) secretion, and LH is required for the formation and maintenance of the corpus luteum and secretion of its hormones, including progesterone. Hormonal patterns during the menstrual cycle are illustrated in Fig. 5-2. The feedback regulation of gonadotropin secretion in women is complex and incompletely understood. Estrogens appear to exert both negative and positive feedback on LH secretion. After a small rise at the end of the preceding luteal phase, LH levels plateau during the follicular phase of the menstrual cycle. This plateau is associated with gradually rising estradiol levels and declining FSH levels. The LH plateau and FSH decline have been attributed to negative feedback by estradiol on gonadotropin secretion. After a major increase in estradiol levels late in the follicular phase, a surge of LH (and FSH) secretion occurs. Ovulation follows the LH peak by less than 24 hours. The mid-cycle LH secretory surge has been attributed to positive feedback by estradiol, perhaps mediated by LH-RH release from the hypothalamus. During the luteal phase of the cycle, estradiol and progesterone levels rise and then fall; LH and FSH levels reach their nadirs and begin to rise again shortly before menstruation begins.

During fetal development, a functioning testis is required for the development of male external and internal genitalia. In the absence of a testis (with or without an ovary), development proceeds along female lines. At puberty, increased gonadotropin se-

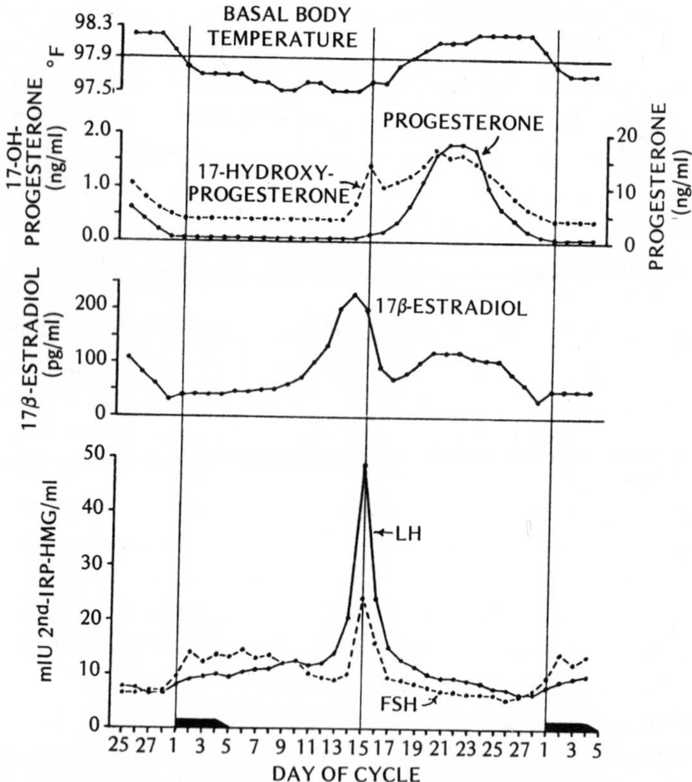

FIG. 5-2. Hormonal patterns during the menstrual cycle. [From Midgley AR Jr, Gay VL, Keyes PL et al, *In* Human Reproduction. Hafez ESE, Evans TN (eds). Harper & Row, Hagerstown, Maryland, 1973, p 201.]

cretion stimulates testicular testosterone secretion, which leads to the development of male secondary sex characteristics, or increased ovarian estrogen secretion, which leads to the development of female secondary sex characteristics. The pubertal increase in sex steroid secretion also triggers a spurt in linear growth followed by epiphyseal fusion and cessation of linear growth. Cyclic gonadotropin secretion at pubertal levels in normal girls leads to the menarche.

ANALYTICAL METHODS

Radioimmunoassays for the measurement of LH, FSH, and testosterone are now rather widely used; specific antisera for estradiol and estrone have been more recently developed. Competitive binding methods, employing corticosteroid binding globulin, have been used for the measurement of progesterone.

Most radioimmunoassays used for the measurement of pituitary gonadotropins lack absolute specificity. For example, antisera against human chorionic gonadotropin (HCG) cross-react with LH and are widely used for the measurement of LH. Since pituitary LH is the predominant circulating species recognized by these antisera, these assays provide an accurate estimate of LH in normal, non-pregnant subjects. Clearly, however, when HCG levels are elevated (as in pregnancy or ectopic HCG secretion), assays of "LH" utilizing these antisera will not accurately reflect pituitary LH secretion. Assays specific for the β-subunit of chorionic gonadotropin (β-HCG) are now available.

In the absence of synthetic LH and FSH standards, the results of LH and FSH assays are expressed in terms of purified LH and FSH extracted from pituitaries or from postmenopausal urine. Since several standards have been used, the interpretation of gonadotropin results requires a knowledge of normal values obtained in the laboratory in which the determinations were performed. Normal serum gonadotropin levels approach the lower limit of sensitivity of many currently available LH and FSH radioimmunoassays. Reported values below the lower limit of sensitivity should not be considered pathologic without evidence of testicular or ovarian failure.

Physiologic variations in gonadotropin levels include episodic secretion, diurnal variation in secretion, and cyclic secretion. Like other pituitary hormones, LH and FSH are secreted in relatively brief bursts. Furthermore, during puberty, circulating gonadotropin levels are higher during sleep than during the waking hours. This observation has been used as an argument for the measurement of LH and FSH in 24-hour urine specimens rather than in random serum samples in adolescents. A more pronounced variation occurs in normally cycling women when serum LH and FSH levels rise several-fold at the time of the mid-cycle surge (Fig. 5-2).

Competitive binding methods, employing sex steroid binding globulin, and radioimmunoassays are used for the measurement of serum testosterone. In the circulation, testosterone is 97 to 99% bound to serum proteins. Like other steroid hormones, the serum testosterone concentration is affected by factors that alter the binding of testosterone to proteins. Factors that increase binding, decrease clearance of testosterone, or both include the presence of high estrogen levels (administered or in pregnancy), cirrhosis, and hyperthyroidism. Factors that decrease binding, increase clearance of testosterone, or both include androgen excess, glucocorticoids, progestins, and hypothyroidism. In women, serum testosterone concentrations vary somewhat during the menstrual cycle, with a nadir in the early follicular phase and a mid-cycle peak. In addition, a diurnal variation in serum testosterone levels, with a morning peak and an evening nadir, has been described in men. Low total serum testosterone levels, without a corresponding reduction in free testosterone levels, have been observed in massively obese men.

Initially, radioimmunoassays for serum estrogens were hampered by a lack of specificity, which necessitated chromatographic isolation of specific estrogens prior to assay. Recently, however, antisera with sufficient specificity for the measurement of estradiol and estrone without chromatography have been developed. The interpretation of serum estradiol levels requires consideration of the changes in levels that occur during the normal menstrual cycle (Fig. 5-2). For example, with some available estradiol immunoassays, normal follicular phase levels approach the lower limit of assay sensitivity. With such assays, pathologically low estradiol levels cannot be clearly distinguished from normal levels when a single determination is performed.

Age is a critical factor in the interpretation of gonadotropin and sex steroid measurements. In the prepubertal period (excluding the postnatal period), all values are low. The decline in estrogen secretion and increase in gonadotropin secretion that are typical of the menopause in women are well known. More recently, a decline in testicular function with advancing age in overtly normal men has been documented. Subtle increases in gonadotropin levels and decreases in the free testosterone concentrations have been found in some men over 40. Frankly elevated gonadotropin levels and low total testosterone concentrations have been found in as many as 30% of men over 70.

Chromosome analysis is often indicated in the evaluation of patients with hypogonadism or ambiguous genitalia. Although determination of the actual chromosomal composition (karyotype) in leukocytes (ideally in multiple tissues including the gonads) is the definitive procedure, a useful screening maneuver for sex chromosome abnormalities is the buccal smear. Normal women (XX) have visible Barr bodies (inactivated X-chromosomes) in more than 20% of buccal epithelial cells (chromatin positive); Barr bodies are not seen (chromatin negative) in buccal epithelial cells from normal men (XY). The buccal smear is a relatively simple screening test, but it is best performed by someone experienced in obtaining, handling, and interpreting the sample.

Semen analysis, including a sperm count and an estimate of the normalcy of sperm morphology and motility, is useful in the evaluation of male infertility. Normal sperm counts are generally greater than 40 million/ml. An adequate sample for semen analysis must be fresh and uncontaminated, i.e., it must be obtained by masturbation into a clean container and transported promptly to the laboratory. Sexual abstinence for 72 hours prior to obtaining the specimen is generally recommended. The entire specimen should be collected, since the majority of the sperm may be concentrated in the initial portion of the ejaculate. Although azoospermic patients are predictably infertile, some patients with distinctly low sperm counts have been fertile. Such factors as sperm motility and morphology and the volume and viscosity of the semen, as well as the absolute sperm count, appear to play important roles in fertility.

Estrogens cause thickening of the vaginal epithelium; the more superficial cells become cornified with pyknotic nuclei. Examination of vaginal smears has been widely used to estimate the presence or absence of normal estrogen levels.

DISORDERS OF GONADAL FUNCTION

DEFICIENT PRODUCTION OF SEX STERIODS The term hypogonadism is most often used to indicate a deficient production of sex steroids by the gonads, usually associated with decreased gamete production. Clearly, infertility can result from deficient gamete production in the absence of recognized abnormalities in sex steroid secretion.

In general, hypogonadism can be primary, due to testicular or ovarian disease, or secondary, due to hypothalamic-pituitary disease. Patients with primary hypogonadism have low levels of the appropriate sex steroids (testosterone or estradiol) and elevated gonadotropin levels. Patients with secondary hypogonadism have low levels of sex steroids without elevation of the gonadotropins. Theoretically, patients with hypothalamic disease should have a normal gonadotropin response to exogenously administered LH-RH, whereas patients with pituitary disease should have no response to LH-RH (analogous to the TSH response to TRH in patients with hypothalamic or pituitary hypothyroidism). Although the frequency of gonadotropin responses to LH-RH can be increased by prolonged LH-RH infusions, many patients with presumed hypothalamic hypogonadism have failed to respond to LH-RH. Nonetheless, an LH and FSH response to LH-RH does provide useful information. The clinical role of other provocative tests, such as the gonadotropin response to clomiphene and the sex steroid response to chorionic gonadotropin, in the detection of incomplete hypogonadism, also remains to be clarified.

MALE HYPOGONADISM Clinically, male hypogonadism is characterized by small testes, absence or regression of secondary sexual characteristics, and often, gynecomastia. The normal adult testis is greater than 3.5 cm in its longest dimension. With practice, the testicular volume can be estimated by palpating the testis with one hand and testicular models of known volume with the other hand. The normal adult testicular volume is approximately 14 to 20 ml, as determined by this method. When testosterone secretion is deficient preceding the usual time of puberty, the clinical appearance is usually easily recognized. The patient will have an infantile penis and scrotum, little or no facial and body hair, and a eunuchoid habitus (including an arm-span more than 2 inches greater than the height), along with small testes. The clinical expression of deficient testosterone secretion that develops after normal pubescence may be more subtle. Diminution in the rate of beard growth, testicular atrophy, and gynecomastia are common manifestations.

Although diminished libido is common in men with hypogonadism, hypogonadism is infrequently found in men who complain of "impotence." Normal adult testosterone levels are not requisite to the attainment of an erection. In most impotent men, neurologic and vascular causes of impotence and hormonal causes of decreased libido are not found, and the symptom is credited to psychogenic factors.

Major causes of male hypogonadism are outlined in Table 5-1. The most common form of *primary hypogonadism* in the male is Klinefelter's syndrome. The prevalence of the Klinefelter's genotype (XXY, XXXY, etc.) has been estimated to be approximately 0.2%. Although Klinefelter's syndrome is a congenital disorder, it does not become clinically overt until the time of expected puberty.* The presence of a normal (prepubertal) male phenotype indicates that sufficient testicular function to direct sexual development must have been present during fetal life. Although failure of normal pubescence and infertility are the rule in patients with Klinefelter's syndrome, the disorder may have variable expression. Some patients have had an apparently normal puberty, and a few have been reported to have fathered children. Patients with Kline-

* Careful estimates of testicular volume in young boys with Klinefelter's syndrome have indicated that the testes are slightly smaller than those of normal prepubertal boys.

Table 5-1
Major causes of male hypogonadism

A. Primary Hypogonadism (Hypergonadotropic Hypogonadism)
   1. Congenital
      a. Klinefelter's syndrome (and its variants)
      b. Functional prepubertal castrate syndrome (anorchia)
      c. Idiopathic Leydig cell and/or seminiferous tubule failure
      d. Other
         male pseudohermaphroditism
         male Turner's syndrome
         "XYY" syndrome
   2. Acquired
      a. Infection (mumps, gonorrhea)
      b. Irradiation, chemotherapy
      c. Trauma (including surgical castration)
      d. Chronic renal failure
      e. Hepatic cirrhosis
      f. Myotonic dystrophy
      g. Idiopathic (including multiple target gland failure, ? autoimmune)

B. Secondary Hypogonadism (Hypogonadotropic Hypogonadism)
   1. Congenital
      a. Isolated gonadotropin deficiency
      b. Multiple tropic hormone deficiencies (panhypopituitarism)
   2. Acquired
      a. Neoplasm
      b. Infarction
      c. Infection (e.g., postmeningitis)
      d. Trauma (including surgery)
      e. Infiltrative diseases (e.g., sarcoidosis, hemochromatosis, histiocytosis)
      f. Idiopathic

felter's syndrome past the age of expected puberty typically have small *firm* testes. Patients with Klinefelter's syndrome tend to be tall; this characteristic has been attributed to the primary genetic disorder, rather than hypogonadism, since the arm-span does not exceed the height.

In view of its frequency, Klinefelter's syndrome should be suspected in all men with primary hypogonadism. The majority of patients with Klinefelter's syndrome have chromatin-positive buccal smears (reflecting the supernumerary X chromosome or chromosomes). It could be pragmatically argued that, in a clinically typical patient, a positive buccal smear represents sufficient documentation for diagnosis (although some less common disorders such as an XX male would not be identified) and that determination of the karyotype, which is expensive, is not necessary. On the other hand, a chromatin negative buccal smear clearly does not exclude the diagnosis of Klinefelter's syndrome. The buccal smear can be negative due to technical error, but is more commonly negative (or equivocal) because of mosaicism. The latter is often detectable by karyotype determination on leukocytes; in some instances, karyotypic study of other tissues, such as the testis, is required. Testicular biopsy, of course, also permits histologic study.

In some hypogonadal patients, the testes are not detectable, although a normal prepubertal male phenotype indicates that testes were present during fetal development. This has been called "anorchia" or the functional prepubertal castrate syndrome. The possibility of cryptorchidism should be kept in mind when this diagnosis is considered. In other patients with primary testicular disorders, the cause of Leydig cell and/or seminiferous tubule failure remains unknown.

Other forms of congenital primary hypogonadism are uncommon. Androgen lack, or resistance to the effects of androgens, during fetal development results in male pseudohermaphroditism (genotypic male with ambiguous or frankly female external genitalia). Androgen lack may be due to enzymatic defects in testosterone synthesis. Androgen resistance may be partial or complete, and it is believed to cause a spectrum of disorders ranging from those of phenotypic males with mild hypospadias and incomplete virilization at puberty (Reifenstein's syndrome) to those of phenotypically normal women with scant or absent pubic and axillary hair and no uterus (testicular feminization syndrome). The basis of male pseudohermaphroditism in patients with mixed gonadal dysgenesis (unilateral testis with a fibrous streak on the other side, XO/XY karyotype) is unknown. These patients may exhibit the somatic abnormalities of Turner's syndrome (see below). Virilization occurs at puberty.

Acquired primary testicular disorders in men most often impair seminiferous tubular function and result in infertility, but they may result in deficient testosterone secretion as well. It should be recalled that men with primary testicular disorders causing oligospermia may be infertile but have normal FSH (and LH and testosterone) levels. In some instances, these disorders may ultimately progress to azoospermia with elevated FSH levels (and, even, testosterone deficiency with elevated LH levels), but this progression is not usually predictable.

Physiologic *secondary hypogonadism* characterizes the prepubertal period. Although puberty is generally well established by the age of 15, it is often difficult to exclude the possibility of delayed puberty with confidence in patients under 20 years of age, particularly if collateral findings with predictive power (e.g., a positive buccal smear, anosmia) are not present.

Isolated gonadotropin deficiency is a not uncommon cause of male hypogonadism. When associated with a decreased olfactory capacity, this disorder is often referred to as Kallman's syndrome and appears to be inherited as an autosomal dominant trait. Less commonly, an isolated deficiency of LH (leading to deficient androgen production in a patient with potential fertility, the so-called fertile eunuch) or of FSH (leading to azoospermia in a patient with normal androgen production) has been recognized.

Functionally, the male gonad can be rather completely evaluated by measurements of the serum testosterone, LH, and FSH and by semen analysis. Patients with primary hypogonadism will have low serum testosterone levels and elevated serum LH levels. If there is associated azoospermia, the serum FSH is usually also elevated. Patients with secondary hypogonadism will have low serum testosterone levels (and sperm counts) with inappropriately low serum LH (and FSH) values. Although additional studies, such as skull films and a buccal smear, are often performed routinely in patients with suspected hypogonadism, it may be more appropriate to establish the functional deficit, and to determine whether it is primary or secondary, first, and then proceed to the etiologic mechanism.

In selected men with hypogonadism or infertility, testicular biopsy may be indicated. The biopsy may have predictive power when (prolonged, expensive) gonadotropin therapy of infertility is seriously anticipated. Biopsy is necessary in the uncommon patient in whom testicular chromosome analysis is indicated and has been advocated for the diagnosis of ductal obstruction (azoospermia with normal spermatogenesis on biopsy). Although testicular biopsy can be performed under local anesthesia with relative safety, the procedure is not without risk. In addition to the usual potential surgical complications, a transient decrease in the sperm count has been noted in up to 45% of subjects biopsied.

FEMALE HYPOGONADISM Hypogonadism in women is manifested clinically by absence or regression of secondary sexual characteristics, infertility, and amenorrhea. Estrogen lack from before the time of normal puberty results in a rather easily recognized clinical picture. These patients have infantile external genitalia, absence of the feminine habitus, no breast development, and a thin, non-cornified vaginal epithelium. Acquired hypogonadism in the previously normal woman is most often heralded by amenorrhea; atrophy of the breasts and vaginal epithelium may subsequently become apparent.

Like male hypogonadism, female hypogonadism can be etiologically categorized as primary (ovarian) or secondary (hypothalamic-pituitary). Gonadal dysgenesis is the most common congenital form of *primary ovarian failure*. Typically, these patients have primary amenorrhea and no secondary sexual characteristics (a few have some vaginal bleeding and breast development) and a variety of somatic abnormalities comprising *Turner's syndrome*. Prominent among the somatic abnormalities are short stature, a short, webbed neck with a low hairline, cubitus valgus, and short metacarpals (most often the fourth). Cardiovascular abnormalities, particularly coarctation of the aorta, occur frequently. The majority of patients with gonadal dysgenesis have absent Barr bodies on buccal smear and a 45 XO karyotype. Others have recognizable X-chromosome abnormalities. Mosaicism may explain the occurrence of Turner's syndrome in patients with normal buccal smears. Patients with 46 XX gonadal dysgenesis ("pure gonadal dysgenesis") often lack the somatic abnormalities of Turner's syndrome.

Acquired forms of primary hypogonadism have been less well characterized in women than in men. It seems likely, however, that the disorders listed in Table 5-1 for men could also cause primary hypogonadism in women. As in males, acquired disorders, short of total ovarian destruction, are more likely to impair fertility than to impair sex steroid secretion. The menopause, of course, produces the typical hormonal pattern of acquired primary hypogonadism in the female.

Isolated deficiencies of LH, FSH, or both are a well-recognized cause of *secondary ovarian failure.* Acquired forms of secondary hypogonadism in women include, in addition to the various causes of hypopituitarism common to both men and women, postpartum pituitary necrosis (Sheehan's syndrome) and post-oral contraceptive amenorrhea and infertility. Psychogenic factors, nutritional factors, or both appear to be capable of impairing gonadotropin secretion. For example, amenorrhea not infrequently accompanies severe emotional stress or major weight loss (or gain). Excessive prolactin secretion is often associated with amenorrhea and infertility. In some instances, pharmacologic suppression of prolactin secretion has been associated with return of menses and fertility (see Chapter 2).

Measurement of serum estrogens should greatly simplify the diagnosis of hypogonadism in women. Although normal early follicular phase estrogen levels may be quite low, and may approach the lower limit of sensitivity of some immunoassays, estradiol levels that are repeatedly shown to be lower than normal follicular phase levels, by a sufficiently sensitive assay, are indicative of pathologic hypogonadism. In contrast to estradiol, which is almost exclusively secreted from the ovaries, circulating estrone is largely formed peripherally from androstenedione secreted from the adrenal cortex as well as the ovary. Thus, serum estrone levels are of less value than estradiol levels in the diagnosis of hypogonadism in women.

Patients with primary ovarian failure will have low estrogen levels and elevated levels of circulating gonadotropins. Marked elevations of plasma FSH have been found to be highly correlated with virtual absence of ovarian follicles. In secondary hypogonadism, both serum estrogens and serum gonadotropins will be inappropriately low. At least one patient with primary amenorrhea, immature ovarian follicles, and undetectable serum FSH, and with low estradiol and elevated LH levels, has been recognized. Measurement of only LH and estradiol would have led to the (incorrect) diagnosis of primary hypogonadism rather than the diagnosis of isolated FSH deficiency.

Although frank hypogonadism with overt estrogen deficiency is uncommon in women in the usual reproductive age range, menstrual abnormalities with or without infertility are common. With the currently expanded analytical armanentarium, it is likely that a variety of abnormalities in the temporal regulation of gonadotropin secretion and quantitative abnormalities in gonadotropin secretion, sex steroid secretion, or both will be delineated in these patients. For example, Sherman and Korenman have detected four groups of ovulatory women who have abnormal menstrual cycles, infertility, or both. Patients with long follicular phases (usually in the post-menarchal age group) or short follicular phases (usually in the pre-menopausal age group) are potentially fertile, whereas patients with short luteal phases or "inadequate" (low progesterone) luteal phases are generally infertile.

The differential diagnosis of amenorrhea can be simplified by dividing patients into those who have never menstruated (primary amenorrhea) and those whose menses have ceased (secondary amenorrhea). In patients with primary amenorrhea, congenital atresia of the uterus and vagina and imperforate hymen must be considered and gonadal dysgenesis, which is found in roughly one-third of such patients, must be specifically sought. In contrast, structural abnormalities of the genital tract are uncommon in women with secondary amenorrhea, although posttraumatic uterine synechiae (i.e., following curettage) can cause amenorrhea. Pregnancy must be the first diagnostic consideration, and menopause the second, in patients with secondary amenorrhea. Other relatively common causes of secondary (rarely primary) amenorrhea include drugs (especially following discontinuation of oral contraceptives or progestins), hyperprolactinemic states (Chapter 2), androgen excess (Chapter 4 and below), and abnormalities of thyroid function (Chapter 3) as well as the psychogenic/nutritional factors mentioned earlier.

EXCESS PRODUCTION OF SEX STEROIDS Overproduction of sex steroids is not uncommon. Androgen excess is more often recognized clinically in women, estrogen excess in men.

ESTROGEN EXCESS The most striking clinical feature of chronic estrogen excess in men is gynecomastia. Testicular atrophy may occur.

Gynecomastia is glandular enlargement of the male breasts and cannot be diagnosed on the basis of appearance alone. Palpably enlarged breast tissue must be present, since obesity can produce pendulous breasts in the absence of gynecomastia. Although tumors of the male breast are uncommon, the first decision the physician must make in evaluating a patient with breast enlargement is whether or not breast tumor is a serious diagnostic possibility. If the breast mass is unilateral, irregular, or associated with nipple discharge, tumor should be the first consideration. Admittedly, gynecomastia can be unilateral, but one can question whether the diagnosis of unilateral gynecomastia should be made in the absence of histologic study. Causes of gynecomastia are outlined in Table 5-2.

Operationally, gynecomastia is believed to be due to either absolute estrogen excess or estrogen excess relative to androgen. Although an increasing number of the conditions listed in Table 5-2

Table 5-2
Differential diagnosis of gynecomastia

A. "Physiologic" Gynecomastia
   1. Gynecomastia in the newborn
   2. Adolescent (pubertal) gynecomastia
   3. Gynecomastia of aging

B. Drugs
   1. Testosterone inhibitors–Spironolactone, cyproterone, flutamine
   2. Estrogen or drugs with estrogen activity–digitalis, marijuana, heroin
   3. Gonadotropins
   4. Other drugs–Androgens, cimetadine, tricyclic antidepressants, ethionamide, anti-adrenergic antihypertensives (e.g., reserpine), bulsulfan

C. Hypergonadotropic States
   1. Primary hypogonadism (see Table 5-1)
   2. Ectopic gonadotropin secretion
      a. Malignancies–especially carcinoma of the lung, but also many others
      b. Testicular tumors

D. Increased Estrogen Formation (Aromatization)
   1. Chronic liver disease
   2. Thyrotoxicosis (?hypothyroidism)
   3. Malnutrition→Refeeding

E. Estrogen Hypersecretion–Testicular or Adrenocortical Tumors

F. Androgen Resistance

are being shown to exhibit these hormonal patterns, there are certain notable exceptions. Most prominent among the latter is the gynecomastia sometimes associated with testosterone (or methyltestosterone) administration.

Certain forms of gynecomastia are sufficiently common to be considered normal. These include gynecomastia in the newborn, attributed to estrogens of maternal origin, placental origin, or both, and adolescent or pubertal gynecomastia attributed to the attainment of adult estradiol production rates prior to the attainment of adult testosterone production rates. These are almost universally transient, although adolescent gynecomastia occasionally persists into adulthood. Gynecomastia of aging has been described and attributed to the acquired primary hypogonadism that may occur in aging men, as discussed above. But an effect of coexistent liver disease or drug administration has not been excluded. Indeed, it is the author's opinion that gynecomastia in an elderly man should not be quickly assigned to "aging" and that the other diagnostic possibilities should be carefully considered.

Gynecomastia may be caused by a variety of drugs (see Table 5-2). Spironolactone is one of the more common offenders; although it is listed as an androgen antagonist, large doses of spironolactone have also been shown to decrease testosterone synthesis. Gynecomastia occurs not infrequently in hypergonadotropic states, including primary hypogonadism and ectopic gonadotropin secretion. In many of these disorders, evidence of increased testicular estrogen secretion, in response to elevated gonadotropin levels, has been demonstrated. It should be recalled that HCG will cross-react with LH in many "LH" radioimmunoassays; thus, a specific measurement of chorionic gonadotropin levels (e.g., β-HCG) is required to separate ectopic gonadotropin secretion from increased pituitary LH secretion. Increased extraglandular conversion of precursor steroids to estrogens (aromatization) is an increasingly recognized mechanism of excessive estrogen formation and the resultant gynecomastia. A disproportionate increase in circulating estrone relative to estradiol provides a clue to this mechanism, although kinetic studies are required to establish it. In chronic liver disease, excessive aromatization of such precursors as Δ^4-androstenedione has been attributed to decreased hepatic clearance of the precursors. Similar mechanisms may be operative in the gynecomastia associated with thyrotoxicosis and that associated with refeeding after a period of malnutrition. Rarely, a primary increase in aromatase activity has been recognized.

Estrogen secreting tumors of the testis or adrenal cortex are rare. The former are often palpable, but may not be, and the latter are generally, but not invariably, associated with overproduction of other adrenocortical hormones. Thus, adrenal and testicular venous sampling may be required to document the abnormal estrogen source. Estrogen secreting testicular tumors are more often benign whereas those of the adrenal cortex are more often malignant.

Lastly, gynecomastia occurs in the rare patient with male pseudohermaphroditism, be it due to defective androgen production (Leydig cell hypoplasia or enzymatic defects in testosterone biosynthesis) or to androgen resistance. The latter patients exhibit a broad range of phenotypic expression ranging from mild hypospadias to a normal female phenotype with a blind vaginal pouch and absent or scanty pubic and axillary hair (testicular feminization).

In summary, evaluation of the patient with gynecomastia should include a complete drug history, consideration of potential gonadotropin secreting tumors, and careful palpation of the abdomen and testes. Chemical studies of hepatic and renal function and basic hormonal measurements, including the serum LH, β-HCG, testosterone, estradiol, and estrone levels and the serum thyroxine concentration, are in order. Clear-cut evidence of unexplained estrogen overproduction should prompt radiographic examination of the adrenal beds (e.g., CT scans of the adrenals), evaluation of the production of adrenocortical hormones, and if necessary, adrenal and testicular vein catheterization.

Estrogen excess in the adult woman is not easily recognized but may produce menstrual abnormalities or post-menopausal vaginal bleeding. In addition to the disorders outlined above, estrogen excess in women has been observed in patients with cancer that has metastasized to the ovaries.

ANDROGEN EXCESS Androgen overproduction in women is discussed in Chapter 4. In general, androgen excess causing acne, hirsutism, and amenorrhea—or more clear-cut virilization with clitoral enlargement, temporal balding, deepening of the voice, and an increase in muscle mass—can be due to either adrenal or ovarian androgen overproduction.

Adrenal androgen overproduction occurs in patients with

Cushing's syndrome, certain enzymatic defects in cortisol synthesis (adrenogenital syndromes), and androgen-secreting adrenocortical tumors. The traditional biochemical marker for adrenal androgen overproduction has been the distinct elevation of the urinary 17-ketosteroids, which are principally derived from adrenal DHA and its metabolites. Recently, however, a few patients with androgen-secreting tumors anatomically located within the adrenal cortex but functionally resembling ovarian tissue (i.e., responsive to gonadotropins) have been recognized. These apparently rare patients have normal base-line 17-ketosteroid excretion.

Ovarian androgen overproduction can result from ovarian tumors, polycystic (sclerocystic) ovaries, or ovarian hyperthecosis. The pathogenesis of the latter two syndromes is unknown. Androgen overproduction with normal 17-ketosteroid excretion and a palpable ovarian abnormality have been considered presumptive evidence for an ovarian androgen source. Minor elevation of urinary 17-ketosteroid excretion (usually less than 20 mg/24 hours), however, has been observed in patients with proven ovarian androgen overproduction.

Ovarian and adrenal vein catheterization studies in women with androgen excess (but without distinct elevation of the urinary 17-ketosteroids) have revealed several important observations. First, the ovary is a common source of androgen. Second, in some instances, excessive androgen secretion can arise from both the ovary and the adrenal gland. Third, suppression and stimulation tests appear to be of no value in predicting the androgen source.

The diagnostic approach to women with evidence of androgen overproduction is outlined in Chapter 4.

Androgen overproduction in men is difficult to recognize clinically, although testicular atrophy could occur, but it has been recognized biochemically on rare occasions.

SUGGESTED READING

1. Paulsen CA: The testes. *In* Textbook of Endocrinology, Fifth Edition. Williams RH (ed). Saunders, Philadelphia, 1974, p 323.

2. Ross GT, Vande Wiele RL: The ovaries. *In* Textbook of Endocrinology, Fifth Edition. Williams RH (ed). Saunders, Philadelphia, 1974, p 368.
3. Chan L, O'Malley BW: Mechanism of action of the sex steroid hormones. *N Engl J Med* 294:1322, 1372, and 1430, 1976.
4. Boyar RM, Ramsey J, Chipman J et al: Regulation of gonadotropin secretion in Turner's syndrome. *N Engl J Med* 298:1328, 1978.
5. Stearns EL, MacDonnell JA, Kaufman BJ et al: Declining testicular function with age. *Amer J Med* 57:761, 1974.
6. Glass AR, Swerdloff RS, Bray GA et al: Low serum testosterone and sex-hormone-binding-globulin in massively obese men. *J Clin Endocrinol Metab* 45:1211, 1977.
7. Penny R, Goldstein IP, Frasier SD: Overnight gonadotropin excretion in normal females. *J Clin Endocrinol Metab* 44:780, 1977.
8. Sherman BM, Korenman SG: Hormonal characteristics of the human menstrual cycle throughout reproductive life. *J Clin Invest* 55:699, 1975.
9. McCann SM: Luteinizing-hormone-releasing hormone. *N Engl J Med* 296:797, 1977.
10. Yoshimoto Y, Moridera K, Imura H: Restoration of normal pituitary gonadotropin reserve by administration of leuteinizing-hormone-releasing hormone in patients with hypogonadotropic hypogonadism. *N Engl J Med* 292:242, 1975.
11. Spitz IM, Diamant Y, Rosen E et al: Isolated gonadotropin deficiency. A heterogeneous syndrome. *N Engl J Med* 290:10, 1974.
12. Maroulis GB, Parlow AF, Marshall JR: Isolated follicle stimulating hormone deficiency in man. *Fertil Steril* 28:818, 1977.
13. Root AW, Reiter EO: Evaluation and management of the child with delayed pubertal development. *Fertil Steril* 27:745, 1976.
14. Odell WD, Swerdloff RS: Abnormalities of gonadal function in men. *Clin Endocrinol* 8:149, 1978.
15. Humphrey TJ, Posen S, Casey JH: Klinefelter's syndrome. Experiences with 24 patients. *Med J Aust* 2:779, 1976.
16. Givens JR: Hirsutism and hyperandrogenism. *Adv Intern Med* 21:221, 1976.
17. Kirschner MA, Zucker IR, Jespersen D: Idiopathic hirsutism—an ovarian abnormality. *N Engl J Med* 294:637, 1976.
18. Aiman J, Edman CD, Worley RJ et al: Androgen and estrogen formation in women with ovarian hyperthecosis. *Obstet Gynec* 51:1, 1978.
19. Rebar R, Judd HL, Yen SSC et al: Characterization of the inappropriate gonadotropin secretion in polycystic ovary syndrome. *J Clin Invest* 57:1320, 1976.

20. Stage AH, Grafton WD: Thecomas and granulosa-theca cell tumors of the ovary. An analysis of 51 tumors. *Obstet Gynec* 50: 21, 1977.
21. Gabrilove JL, Nicolis GL, Mitty HL, Sohval AR: Feminizing interstitial cell tumor of the testis: Personal observation and a review of the literature. *Cancer* 35:1184, 1975.
22. Rosen SW, Weintraub BD, Vaitukaitis JL et al: Placental proteins and their subunits as tumor markers. *Ann Intern Med* 82:71, 1975.
23. Wilson JD, MacDonald PC: Male pseudohermaphroditism due to androgen resistance: Testicular feminization and related syndromes. *In* The Metabolic Basis of Inherited Disease. Fourth Edition. Stanburg JB, Wyngaarden JB, Frederickson DS (eds). McGraw-Hill, New York, 1978, p 894.

6

THE ADRENERGIC NERVOUS SYSTEM

Catecholamines are synthesized from tyrosine in neurons of the central and peripheral (sympathetic) nervous systems and in chromaffin cells. Norepinephrine (NE) and its precursor dopamine are synaptic neurotransmitters in the central nervous system. Norepinephrine is also the neurotransmitter released from sympathetic postganglionic neurons of the peripheral nervous system. Epinephrine (E), on the other hand, is a classic hormone in that it is secreted (from the adrenal medulla) into the circulation and produces its metabolic effects at distant sites.

N-Methylation of NE to form E is accomplished in chromaffin cells. Chromaffin cells are widespread and intimately associated with the sympathetic nervous system during fetal life but, for the most part, degenerate postnatally. The major residual clusters of functioning chromaffin cells compose the adrenal medulla. Like the adrenergic postganglionic sympathetic neurons, the chromaffin cells of the adrenal medulla are innervated by cholinergic preganglionic sympathetic neurons.

The structure of NE and certain conventions of catecholamine nomenclature are illustrated in Fig. 6-1. The biosynthesis of catecholamines from tyrosine is outlined in Fig. 6-2. Tyrosine hydroxylase, which catalyzes the hydroxylation of tyrosine to form

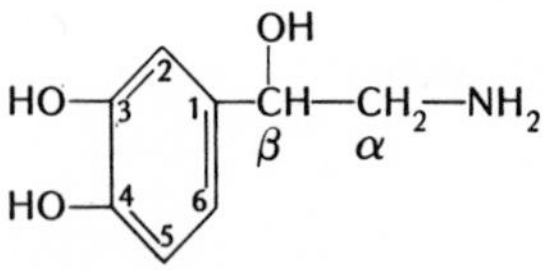
OH
HO
HO
CH—CH2—NH2
β α
1 2 3 4 5 6

FIG 6-1. The structure of norepinephrine and certain conventions of catecholamine nomenclature.

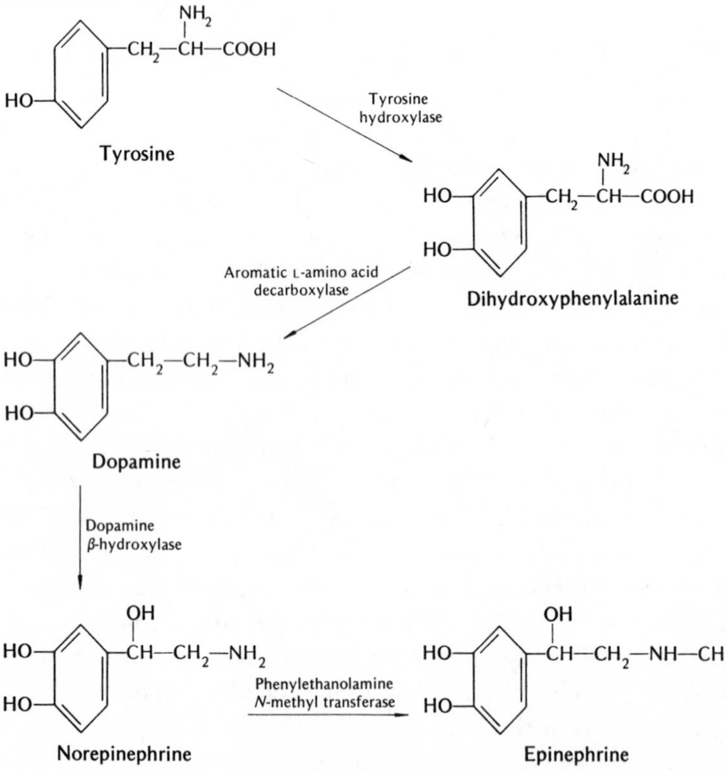
Tyrosine
Tyrosine hydroxylase
Dihydroxyphenylalanine
Aromatic L-amino acid decarboxylase
Dopamine
Dopamine β-hydroxylase
Norepinephrine
Phenylethanolamine N-methyl transferase
Epinephrine

FIG. 6-2. Catecholamine biosynthesis.

dihydroxyphenylalanine (dopa), is the rate limiting enzyme in catecholamine synthesis. Phenylethanolamine *N*-methyl transferase, which converts NE to E, is present in the adrenal medulla. Its persistence in anatomic relation to the adrenal cortex may be due, in part, to the fact that it is a glucocorticoid-inducible enzyme. Nonetheless, E synthesis can occur in chromaffin tissue remote from the adrenal cortex as evidenced by the rare, but well-documented examples of extra-adrenal E-producing pheochromocytomas.

The major routes of catecholamine degradation are illustrated in Fig. 6-3. Catechol-*o*-methyl transferase (COMT), a ubiquitous enzyme, catalyzes methylation of the hydroxyl group at C_3 of the catecholamine ring, thus converting NE and E to biologically

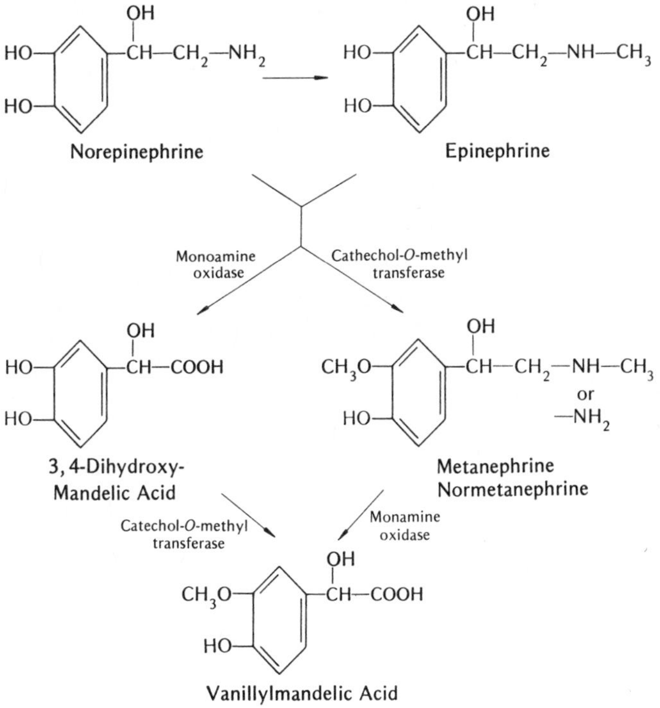

FIG. 6-3. Catecholamine metabolism.

inactive metabolites, normetanephrine (NMN) and metanephrine (MN), and converting the oxidized catecholamine metabolite, 3,4-dihydroxymandelic acid, to the major end product of catecholamine metabolism, 3-methoxy-4-hydroxymandelic acid, better known as vanillylmandelic acid (VMA). The monoamine oxidases (MAO) are mitochondrial enzymes that oxidize the catecholamines to 3,4-dihydroxymandelic acid (also biologically inactive) and NMN or MN to VMA.*

Homovanillic acid (HVA), not illustrated in Fig. 6-3, is the major oxidized and *o*-methylated derivative of dopamine. The structure of HVA is identical to that of VMA, except HVA lacks a hydroxyl group on the beta-carbon.

A highly schematic overview of the physiology of the adrenergic axon terminal is shown in Fig. 6-4. Tyrosine is transported into mitochondria of the adrenergic axon terminal where it is hydroxylated to dopa. In the cytoplasm, dopa is decarboxylated to dopamine. Beta-hydroxylation of dopamine to NE occurs within "storage" (or "secretion") granules, where NE is protected from the intraneuronal mitochondrial monoamine oxidases. Upon depolarization of the axon, a bolus of NE is released into the synaptic cleft where it gains access to receptor sites on the effector cell. Release of granule contents into the synaptic cleft is thought to occur by exocytosis, i.e., migration of the granule to the plasma membrane of the axon terminal, fusion of the adjacent granule and terminal membranes, with subsequent dissolution of the fused membranes, and release of the entire granule contents into the synaptic cleft.

There are three major routes of biologic inactivation of released NE:

1. Reuptake into the axon terminal (the major route).
2. Local enzymatic degradation.
3. Escape into the circulation.

* This is the "oxidative pathway" of catcholamine degradation. The end product of the "reductive pathway," 3-methoxy-4-hydroxyphenylglycol, is believed to be the major metabolite of NE in the central nervous system.

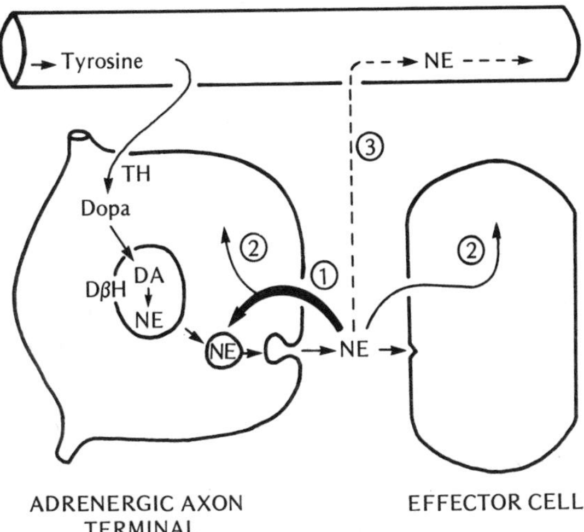

FIG. 6-4. Overview of norepinephrine synthesis, storage, release, reuptake, local metabolism, and escape into the circulation.

The NE and E that enter the circulation are largely metabolized by MAO and COMT in the liver. Thus, under usual circumstances, only microgram quantities of NE and E appear in a 24-hour urine specimen, whereas milligram quantities of catecholamine metabolites, such as VMA, are excreted in the urine.

Since the vast bulk of released NE is dissipated by reuptake and local metabolism, plasma NE represents only a small fraction of released NE. Thus, a steep NE gradient exists between the synaptic cleft and the plasma. From this, one would expect that if NE were introduced directly into circulation, very high plasma levels would be required to produce biologically effective synaptic cleft NE concentrations.

Catecholamines modulate not only traditional gross physiologic (heart rate, bronchiolar tone, gastrointestinal motility, etc.) and metabolic (lipolysis, glycogenolysis, gluconeogenesis, etc.) events but also the secretion of a variety of hormones. The full range of catcholamine effects is exhibited during the massive adrenergic discharge precipitated by severe stress, as summarized in Table

6-1. It is reasonable to suspect that NE-mediated adrenergic modulation is also involved in the maintenance of metabolic homeostasis in the non-stressed state.

Catecholamines interact with membrane-bound cellular receptors as an initial step in hormone action. At least two types of adrenergic receptors (alpha and beta) have been recognized, and they are operationally defined on the basis of studies with various adrenergic agonists and blocking agents (see Table 6-1). Although certain drugs produce relatively pure alpha- (phenylephrine, methoxamine) or beta- (isoproterenol) adrenergic stimulation, the endogenous catecholamines, NE and E, can interact with both alpha- and beta-adrenergic receptors. Thus, the response of a given cell to catecholamines is a function of the type of receptors that populates that cell as well as the particular catecholamine presented to that cell. For example, the intravenous infusion of NE produces a response typical of alpha-adrenergic stimulation (increased peripheral resistance with a rise in the blood pressure and a reflex reduction in cardiac rate and output); this indicates that NE is a more potent alpha- than beta-adrenergic stimulator. On the other hand, NE released from axon terminals within the myocardium produces a pattern of beta-adrenergic stimulation (increased cardiac rate and output), since the myocardium is populated by beta receptors.

As a generalization, the cellular response to beta-adrenergic stimulation is mediated via adenylate cyclase stimulation and generation of intracellular cyclic AMP (cAMP). The relationship between alpha-adrenergic stimulation and the "second messenger" system is not, as yet, established. In some instances, alpha stimulation lowers intracellular cAMP levels; this implies inhibition of adenylate cyclase.

ANALYTICAL METHODS

Catecholamines are routinely measured fluorometrically. Free catecholamines are extracted from urine and oxidized to their more intensely fluorescent trihydroxyindole derivatives. Tech-

Table 6-1
Catecholamine effects

	ALPHA	BETA
Hormonal secretion[a]		
Pancreas	Decreased insulin secretion	Increased glucagon secretion[b]
Pituitary	Increased growth hormone secretion Increased ACTH secretion	
Kidney		Increased renin secretion
Metabolic changes		
Fat		Lipolysis, free fatty acid release
Muscle		Glycolysis, lactate release
Liver	Glycogenolysis, gluconeogenesis, glucose release[b]	
Functional changes		
Arterioles	Constriction	Dilation (especially in skeletal muscle)
Heart		Increased rate and force of ventricular contraction
Bronchioles		Dilation
Gastrointestinal tract	Decreased motility	Decreased motility
Sweat glands	Increased sweating (especially of palms)	
Pupils	Mydriasis	

[a] Adrenergic mechanisms may modulate the secretion of other hormones, e.g., LH, FSH, vasopressin, thyroid hormones, and parathyroid hormone.
[b] Available data concerning the assignment of increased hormone secretion to alpha- or beta-adrenergic mechanisms are contradictory.

nical maneuvers (reading at two different wavelengths, performance of the oxidation at two pH levels) permit fractionation of the catecholamines into NE and E.*

Fluorometric catecholamine assays have been applied to plasma as well as urine. These methods are adequate for the measurement of catecholamines in urine, where the concentrations are up to 100-fold higher than in plasma. With respect to plasma, however, their limited sensitivity makes them inadequate for measurement of variations within the physiologic range or for detection of minor elevations. Recently, enzymatic isotope-derivative methods for the measurement of NE and E have been developed. These are based upon the conversion of NE and E to labeled NMN and labeled MN when the catecholamines are incubated with S-adenosylmethionine containing a labeled methyl group in the presence of catechol-*o*-methyl transferase. These methods provide the requisite sensitivity and precision for measurement of NE and E in plasma, but are complex, time consuming, and relatively expensive. Nonetheless, one such assay is now commercially available.

Urinary normetanephrine plus metanephrine ("total metanephrines") and vanillylmandelic acid (VMA) are selectively extracted from urine and converted to vanillin, which is then measured spectrophotometrically.

Although technically demanding, these determinations can be performed with acceptable precision (i.e., coefficient of variation of replicate determinations of catecholamines from the same urine sample in serial assays less than 10% by an experienced laboratory technician). Although analytical error can be a cause of di-

* These separations of NE and E are not complete. For example, at pH 7.0, both NE and E are oxidized, but at pH 2.0, E is the predominant catecholamine oxidized. Nonetheless, approximately 5 to 10% of the fluorescence developed after oxidation at pH 2.0 is derived from NE (Anton and Sayre). Therefore, when the concentration of NE greatly exceeds that of E in the sample (in the urine the ratio is approximately 10 : 1) an appreciable fraction of the reported E will actually reflect NE. A 24-hour urine collection reported to contain 100 μg of NE and 5 to 10 μg of E may, in fact, contain no E whatsoever.

agnostic confusion, particularly in laboratories in which these measurements are performed infrequently, such confusion more often arises from errors in urine collection, collection of specimens during major stress, or the administration of medications that alter the physiology or affect the analysis of catecholamines, their metabolites, or both.

The collection of a complete 24-hour urine specimen requires careful instruction of both the patient and the nursing staff, as noted previously. The creatinine content should be measured in all specimens to determine if major collection errors have occurred. These maneuvers are discussed at greater length in Chapter 4.

Although routine activity need not be limited, major stress must be avoided during urine collection. For example, performance of an aortogram can produce a two- to threefold increase in 24-hour catecholamine excretion.

A large variety of drugs alter catecholamine physiology and, thus, have the potential to distort urinary determinations of catecholamines. Other medications interfere directly with the analytical techniques. The effects of medication on urinary catecholamines, NMN and MN, and VMA are summarized in Table 6-2.

Drug-induced elevation of measured urinary catecholamines due to analytical artifact is often recognized in the laboratory. For example, patients ingesting fluorescent drugs, such as tetracycline, will have elevated urinary "catecholamines" measured fluorometrically. Here, excessive fluorescence in urine-containing blanks will also be present and should alert the laboratory staff to the presence of drug-induced artifact. Major diagnostic confusion more often occurs when increased catecholamine excretion is due to drugs that are catecholamines or that alter catecholamine metabolism. Inhaled catecholamines (including isoproterenol), nasal vasoconstrictors, and ingested catecholamine releasing drugs (such as ephedrine, methylxanthines, and amphetamines) are common offenders. Chronic L-dopa therapy elevates VMA excretion without major changes in NE or E excretion. Alpha-methyldopa is metabolized to alpha-methylnorepinephrine and alpha-methyl-

Table 6-2

Medication-induced alterations in the measurement of catecholamines, total metanephrines, and vanillylmandelic acid

INCREASE

CATECHOLAMINES	NMN	VMA
Catecholamines	Catecholamines	Catecholamines
Alpha-methyldopa	Alpha-methyldopa	
MAO inhibitors	MAO inhibitors	
Ephedrine	Ephedrine	Ephedrine
Amphetamines	Amphetamines	Amphetamines
Methylxanthines	Methylxanthines	Methylxanthines
Nitroglycerin	Nitroglycerin	Nitroglycerin
Phenothiazines[a]	Phenothiazines[a]	Phenothiazines[a]
Tricyclic antidepressants[a]	Tricyclic antidepressants[a]	Tricyclic antidepressants[a]
Tetracycline		Nalidixic acid
Erythromycin		Para-aminosalicyclic acid (PAS)
Methenimine		Bromosulfophthalein (BSP)
Mandelamine		Phenolsulfophthalein (PSP)
Chloral hydrate		
Quinidine		
Quinine		
Bretylium		
Methocarbamol		
Bromosulfophthalein (BSP)		
Phenolsulfophthalein (PSP)		
Methylphenidate		
Nicotinic acid		
Riboflavin		

DECREASE

CATECHOLAMINES	NMN	VMA
Alpha-methyl-para-tyrosine	Alpha-methyl-para-tyrosine	Alpha-methyl-para-tyrosine
Clonidine	Clonidine	Clonidine

Table 6-2 Continued

Reserpine	Reserpine	Reserpine
Guanethidine	Guanethidine	Guanethidine
Guanoxan	Guanoxan	Guanoxan
		MAO inhibitors
		Clofibrate
		Mandelamine

[a] Acute effect. Chronic therapy may decrease catecholamine excretion.

normetanephrine, which are measured in the catecholamine and total metanephrine determinations, respectively.* These compounds cannot serve as substrates for MAO; therefore, VMA excretion is not altered. Monoamine oxidase inhibitors increase catecholamine and total MN excretion modestly (and decrease VMA excretion). Additional drugs causing an elevation in catecholamine excretion are listed in Table 6-2.

Artifactual depression of catecholamine excretion is a potential diagnostic problem. Chronic therapy with such agents as reserpine and guanethidine produces small decreases in the excretion of catecholamines and their metabolites. Although it is unlikely that the magnitude of this effect would be great enough to obscure the diagnosis of most pheochromocytomas, difficulty might conceivably arise in a patient with marginally elevated urine values initially. In contrast, alpha-methyl-paratyrosine, a tyrosine hydroxylase inhibitor used experimentally in the therapy of unresectable pheochromocytomas, regularly lowers the excretion of catecholamines and their metabolites. The ingestion of MAO inhibitors depresses VMA excretion in normal subjects and represents a potential problem in a patient with a pheochromocytoma that releases relatively small amounts of catecholamines. Hydralazine does not alter catecholamine excretion nor does chronic thiazide therapy. Clonidine, a new antihypertensive agent, reduces sympathetic activity and has been reported to lower plasma and

* These determinations can be performed 72 hours after alpha-methyldopa is discontinued.

urine catecholamine levels. One would not expect clonidine to lower catecholamine excretion greatly in patients with pheochromocytomas, although data on this point are lacking.

Clearly, it is preferable to withhold all medications during the measurement of urinary catecholamines and their metabolites. On the other hand, the short-term administration of mild analgesics (such as acetylsalicylic acid, acetaminophen, and propoxyphene) and of mild sedatives and tranquilizers (such as phenobarbital, diphenhydramine, chlordiazepoxide, and diazepam) in the usual dosages does not alter catecholamine excretion.

DISORDERS OF THE ADRENERGIC NERVOUS SYSTEM

The only well-established disorder of *catecholamine excess* is hypertension as the result of catecholamine secretion from tumors arising from chromaffin tissues, *pheochromocytomas.* Excessive adrenergic activity, however, may play a role in a variety of disorders. For example, there is renewed interest in the study of catecholamines in essential hypertension. The possibility that adrenergic mechanisms contribute to the pathogenesis of hormonal disorders, such as the impaired insulin secretion in diabetes and the excessive secretion of growth hormone in acromegaly, has been raised.

Only one hypertensive patient in 200 harbors a pheochromocytoma. But, this form of secondary hypertension is particularly important to detect since:

1. The hypertension is often surgically curable.
2. The patient with a pheochromocytoma is continuously at risk for a lethal hypertensive paroxysm.
3. There is an incidence of malignancy (approximately 5%) among pheochromocytomas.
4. The presence of a pheochromocytoma is a diagnostic clue to the presence of associated neuroectodermal or endocrine diseases and raises the possibility of a familial disorder.

Roughly one-half the patients with pheochromocytomas have intermittent hypertension. The remainder have persistent hypertension, often with marked fluctuations in blood pressure. Paroxysmal hypertension and paroxysmal symptoms (especially bouts of severe headache associated with diaphoresis and palpitations) are highly suggestive of pheochromocytoma. In large series, approximately three-fourths of the patients with recognized pheochromocytomas have had such paroxysmal symptoms. This represents a selected group of patients, however. The frequency of typical symptoms would be expected to be considerably lower among patients discovered by routine screening of a large hypertensive population. Episodes of hypotension, tachycardia, and fever raise the possibility of a pheochromocytoma that predominantly secretes E, which is uncommon.

The preoperative diagnosis of a pheochromocytoma is a biochemical one. Clinical features, responses to pharmacologic tests, and anatomic (usually radiographic) evidence of an adrenal tumor are only suggestive.

Many endocrinologists routinely use the measurement of catecholamines, total metanephrines (NMN plus MN), and/or VMA in a 24-hour urine collection as both a screening and a definitive test for the diagnosis of pheochromocytoma. Others, including some who have extensive experience with this disease, use spot urines rather than 24-hour collections. In this test, the VMA (or total metanephrines) and creatinine are measured in an untimed urine specimen, and the results are expressed in milligrams per gram of creatinine. Using this form of expression, Gitlow found urinary VMA levels of greater than 5 mg/gm creatinine in all but 3 of 92 patients with pheochromocytomas and less than 5 mg/gm creatinine in over 9500 (noncomatose) patients without pheochromocytomas.

Although determinations performed on spot urines may be acceptable for screening purposes, the measurement of catecholamines and VMA and/or total metanephrines in a complete 24-hour urine collection is preferable for the diagnosis of a pheochromocytoma. Fractionation of the catecholamines, with determination of NE and E excretion, is indicated when clinical features suggest predominant E secretion by the tumor. As illustrated in Fig. 6-5, 24-hour urinary catecholamines, VMA, and total meta-

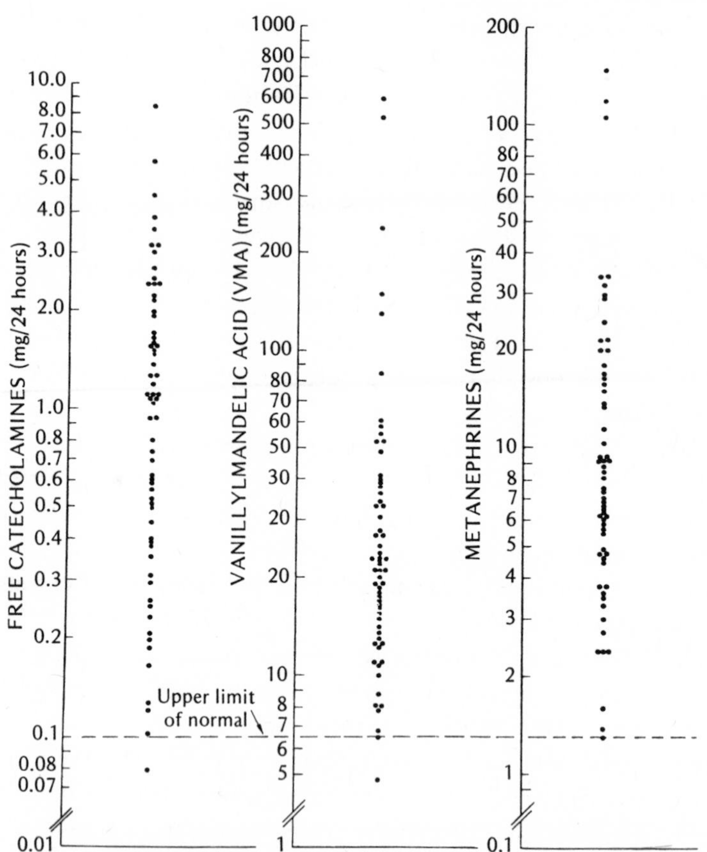

FIG. 6-5. The 24-hour urinary excretion of catecholamines, vanillylmandelic acid (VMA), and total metanephrines in 64 patients with pheochromocytoma (note the log scales). (From Sjoerdsma A, Engelman K, Waldman TA et al: *Am Int Med* 65:1302, 1966.)

nephrines are distinctly elevated in the majority of patients with pheochromocytomas. Thus, if the excretion of catecholamines and their metabolites is clearly normal in two accurately collected 24-hour urines, pheochromocytoma is unlikely. If the clinical picture is highly suggestive, the patient should be reevaluated in the future.

In the majority of patients with pheochromocytomas, the only clinical manifestations of the tumor are those caused by catecholamines released from the tumor into the circulation. As mentioned earlier, very high plasma NE concentrations are required to produce biologically effective NE concentrations within the synaptic clefts. Thus, one would expect that patients with clinically apparent pheochromocytomas would have markedly elevated plasma NE levels. The author's experience with isotope-derivative measurements of plasma NE and E concentrations in 13 patients with surgically proven pheochromocytomas is summarized in Fig. 6-6. All samples were drawn with the patients in the basal state and supine position; sampling during symptomatic paroxysms was specifically avoided. Plasma NE levels were elevated, often markedly so, in 12 of the patients. Patient number 12, with a normal plasma NE level at the time of sampling, was also normotensive at that time. Although the plasma E level was elevated in the latter patient, E levels were normal on at least one occasion in six of the patients. The clinical picture in patient number 13, with the highest basal plasma E concentrations, was dominated by episodes of hypotension typical of a predominantly E secreting pheochromocytoma.

Pharmacologic tests have been devised for the diagnosis of pheochromocytoma. These tests are potentially dangerous and have approximately a 25% incidence of false positives and false negatives. With the availability of accurate methods for the measurement of catecholamines and their metabolites, these tests are rarely, if ever, indicated.

Two types of pharmacologic tests have been used in the past. In patients with sustained hypertension due to a pheochromocytoma, the diastolic blood pressure usually falls more than 25 mm Hg a few minutes after the intravenous injection of the alpha-adrenergic blocking agent phentolamine (Regitine). If a Regitine test is to be performed, a test dose of 0.5 to 1.0 mg should be tried initially, since the often recommended dose of 5.0 mg may produce severe hypotension in a patient with a pheochromocytoma. Provocative tests (histamine, tyramine, glucagon) have been devised for patients with intermittent hypertension. For example,

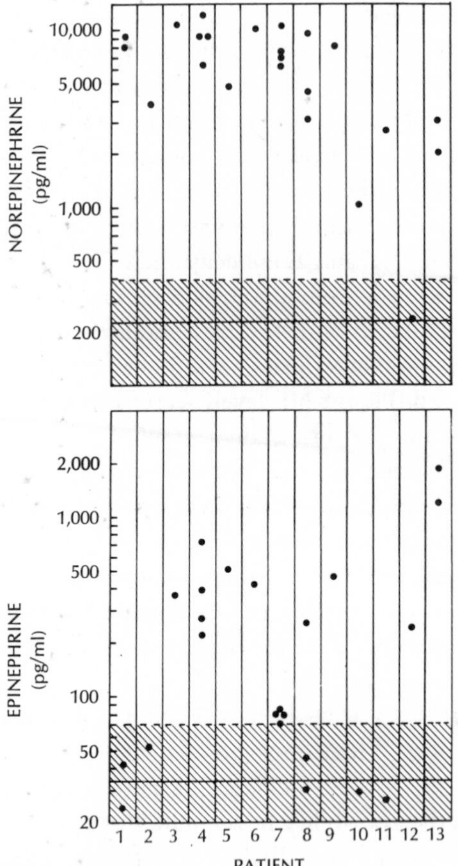

FIG. 6-6. Basal plasma norepinephrine and epinephrine concentrations in 13 patients with surgically proven pheochromocytomas. Note the log scales. The interrupted horizontal line is two standard derivations above the mean (solid horizontal line) values from 60 normal subjects.

intravenous glucagon (1.0 mg administered during a normotensive interval) may result in a sharp increase in the blood pressure in a patient with a pheochromocytoma. If a provocative test is performed, an intravenous line should be established for the injection of phentolamine (5.0 mg) if it is necessary to abort a severe hypertensive paroxysm, which may occur in patients with pheochromocytomas. Before performing any of these pharmacologic tests the physician must ask himself "Will I recommend surgery if the provocative test is positive and the catecholamine determinations are consistently normal?" If the answer is no, the risks of the pharmacologic tests are difficult to justify.

Although pheochromocytomas have arisen from chromaffin cells in locations ranging from the carotid body to the urinary bladder, 98% are within the abdomen (especially in the adrenal medulla), and most of the remainder are in the posterior mediastinum. Thus, physical examination and chest films with oblique views constitute adequate preoperative tumor localization in the patient with convincing clinical and biochemical evidence of a pheochromocytoma. Computed tomographic scans may demonstrate an adrenal tumor. In view of the 10 to 20% incidence of multiple pheochromocytomas, however, the surgeon is no less obligated to explore the abdomen thoroughly by the preoperative demonstration of an adrenal tumor. Therefore, arteriography, with its attendant risks, is not routinely recommended. If it is decided to do an arteriogram on a patient with clinical and biochemical evidence of a pheochromocytoma, it should be done only after the establishment of adequate alpha-adrenergic blockade with phenoxybenzamine as evidenced by control of the blood pressure and prevention of paroxysms.

The conditions sometimes associated with pheochromocytomas —neurofibromatosis, angiomatosis of the retina and cerebellum, (von Hippel-Lindau), neurofibromatosis, and multiple endocrine neoplasia, type 2 (medullary carcinoma of the thyroid, hyperparathyroidism, and pheochromocytoma)—should be kept in mind during diagnostic evaluation of a patient with a pheochromocytoma. Several instances of familial pheochromocytoma (including the multiple endocrine neoplasia, type 2 syndrome) have been documented. Interestingly, the incidence of bilateral pheochromocytoma exceeds 50% in patients with this autosomal dominant disorder.

Clinical and biochemical evidence of *adrenergic insufficiency* is exhibited in the syndrome of *primary autonomic dysfunction*. Patients with this syndrome have various symptoms and signs of disease involving the autonomic nervous system including postural hypotension, impaired sweating, impotence, and at times, abnormalities of bladder and rectal sphincter function. In contrast to patients with postural hypotension due to intravascular volume contraction or decreased cardiac and/or arteriolar responsiveness to NE (e.g., glucocorticoid lack), patients with postural hypotension due to autonomic dysfunction are characterized clinically by the absence of an appropriate postural increase in the pulse rate. It has recently been demonstrated that the normal postural increase in plasma NE is absent or markedly blunted in such patients. A similar plasma catecholamine pattern has been described in patients with autonomic neuropathy associated with diabetes.

SUGGESTED READING

1. Cryer PE: Diseases of the adrenal medullae and sympathetic nervous system. *In* Endocrinology and Metabolism. Felig P, Baxter J, Broadus A, Frohman L (eds). McGraw-Hill, New York, In Press.
2. Cryer PE: Isotope derivative measurements of plasma norepinephrine and epinephrine in man. *Diabetes* 25:1071, 1976.
3. Silverberg AB, Shah SD, Haymond MW, Cryer PE: Norepinephrine: Hormone and neurotransmitter in man. *Amer J Physiol* 234:E252, 1978.
4. Manger WM, Gifford RW: Current concepts of pheochromocytoma. *Cardiovasc Med* 3:289, 1978.
5. Gitlow SE, Mendlowitz M, Bertani LM: The biochemical techniques for detecting and establishing the presence of a pheochromocytoma. *Amer J Cardiol* 26:270, 1970.
6. Steiner AL, Goodman AD, Powers SR: Study of a kindred with pheochromocytoma, medullary thyroid carcinoma, hyperparathyroidism and Cushing's disease: Multiple endocrine neoplasia, type 2. *Medicine* 47:371, 1968.
7. Cryer PE, Weiss S: Reduced plasma norepinephrine response to standing in autonomic dysfunction. *Arch Neurol* 33:275, 1976.

7

THE PARATHYROIDS AND VITAMIN D

Parathyroid hormone (PTH) stimulates resorption of calcium and phosphate from bone, calcium reabsorption and phosphate excretion by the kidneys, and directly or indirectly, absorption of calcium and phosphate from the gastrointestinal tract. The major effect of vitamin D is to stimulate calcium and phosphate absorption from the gastrointestinal tract, although vitamin D may also have direct effects on calcium and phosphate deposition in bone and reabsorption by the kidneys.

The major determinant of PTH secretion is the extracellular calcium concentration. In the circulation, calcium is partially bound to serum proteins. A fall in the free calcium concentration triggers PTH secretion, a rise suppresses PTH secretion. The effects of changes in the serum phosphate concentration on PTH secretion are thought to be indirect and to be due to reciprocal changes in the serum free calcium level. Acute hypomagnesemia also triggers PTH secretion. But at least in organ culture systems, a great reduction in the extracellular magnesium concentration results in suppressed PTH secretion. Beta-adrenergic stimulation of PTH secretion has been demonstrated, but the physiologic role of the autonomic nervous system, if any, in the regulation of PTH secretion remains to be established.

The biologic effects of PTH are believed to be mediated, at

least in part, through activation of adenylate cyclase in target tissues. The administration of exogenous PTH causes a sharp increase in urinary cAMP excretion.

Vitamin D is derived from the diet (largely ergocalciferol, vitamin D_2) or from cutaneous conversion of 7-dehydrocholecalciferol to cholecalciferol (vitamin D_3) upon exposure to ultraviolet light. Vitamin D is stored in fat and is bound to an alpha-globulin in the circulation. It is rather rapidly removed from the circulation (plasma half-time approximately 24 hours) by the liver where the parent vitamin is hydroxylated to form 25-hydroxyvitamin D (25-OHD), which is further hydroxylated in the kidneys to form 1,25-dihydroxyvitamin D [1,25-$(OH)_2D$]. The latter, 1,25-$(OH)_2D$, is the most potent vitamin D metabolite known and may well be the physiologic form of vitamin D. In contrast to 25-hydroxylation, further hydroxylations occur more slowly; the plasma half-time of 25-OHD is 7 to 14 days. Regulation of renal 1-hydroxylation of 25-OHD to form 1,25-$(OH)_2D$ may provide control of the metabolic effects of vitamin D. Factors that favor formation of 1,25-$(OH)_2D$ include low calcium and phosphorous levels and high PTH levels.

Calcitonin (thyrocalcitonin) is a hypocalcemic hormone, secreted predominantly from thyroid parafollicular cells (C-cells) in response to hypercalcemia. Its principal effect is to inhibit bone resorption; it may also impair calcium absorption from the gastrointestinal tract and reabsorption from the renal tubules.

Bone is a metabolically active tissue that undergoes continuous remodeling (old bone resorption and new bone formation) throughout life. The maximal bone mass is achieved in the mid-thirties; thereafter resorption exceeds formation, and the bone mass gradually declines. Multiple humoral factors [principally PTH and 1,25-$(OH)_2D$ but also sex steroids, glucocorticoids, thyroid hormones, growth hormone, and perhaps calcitonin] participate in the regulation of the formation and resorption of bone.

Calcium is not only a major structural component of bone, it is critical to a variety of biochemical processes including those underlying muscle contraction and nerve conduction and the secretion of several hormones.

ANALYTICAL METHODS

The development of radioimmunoassays for PTH in serum has not only stimulated research into the physiology and pathophysiology of mineral metabolism, but has also facilitated the clinical evaluation of patients with disorders of mineral metabolism. The critical analysis of apparently contradictory findings using different PTH antisera has led to a major clarification of the physiology of PTH secretion and has established precedents for the study of peptide hormones in general. Nonetheless, many questions remain. A number of circulating "fragments" and "prohormones" have been recognized, but for the most part, their origin and physiologic significance remain to be definitely established.

In the clinical interpretation of PTH radioimmunoassays, an awareness of the characteristics of the specific assay system used is particularly critical. Nevertheless, certain generalizations can be made:

1. In the absence of purified human PTH standards, the results of PTH assays are generally expressed in terms of either arbitrary "microliter equivalents" of a hyperparathyroid serum or quantities of purified animal PTH. Thus, normal values cannot be transposed from assay to assay and must be carefully established for each individual assay.

2. Most PTH radioimmunoassays are not sufficiently sensitive to distinguish low values from normal values, i.e., the lower limit of sensitivity lies within the normal range.

3. Many antisera used to measure PTH recognize the carboxy-terminal portion of the molecule and measure biologically inactive molecules with relatively long plasma half-times (hours). It appears that this represents a diagnostic advantage due to the relative stability of the plasma concentration of these molecules. Antisera that recognize the amino-terminal portion of the molecule, including biologically active molecules with relatively short plasma half-times (minutes), have been developed but are not widely available. In general, the latter have been less effective in the diagnosis of hyperparathyroidism.

4. Most antisera used in the radioimmunoassay of PTH cross-react incompletely, if at all, with "ectopic" PTH secreted from nonparathyroid tumors. The use of multiple antisera, however, will increase the yield of measurably elevated PTH levels in such patients.

It has been difficult to develop suitably sensitive radioimmunoassays for calcitonin. But, relatively complex assays capable of measuring calcitonin levels in normal subjects have now been developed and have been applied to the study of calcitonin physiology and pathophysiology, although they are not widely available.

Competitive binding assays for 25-hydroxyvitamin D are available in a few centers. A competitive binding method for the measurement of 1,25-dihydroxyvitamin D has been used and a radioimmunoassay has recently been described. Although experience with these complex assays in clinical diagnosis has been limited, it is reasonable to expect that technical advances will lead to their more widespread availability and clinical utility.

The development of atomic absorption methodology has permitted the precise measurement of total serum calcium concentration. Automated colorimetric methods also give satisfactory results when they are carefully calibrated. In the circulation, calcium is partially bound to serum proteins (chiefly albumin). Thus, changes in the concentration of serum proteins can produce corresponding changes in the total calcium concentration without a change in the free calcium concentration. Although a number of formulas have been devised to estimate the effect of changes in the serum protein levels on the total calcium concentration,* direct measurement of the free ("ionized") calcium concentration, using a calcium-sensitive electrode, is preferable. Samples for free calcium determinations must be handled anaerobically and transported on ice. Magnesium is also measured by an atomic absorption method. Like calcium, magnesium is partially bound to serum proteins in the circulation.

* Perhaps the simplest rule is that a reduction of the serum albumin of 1.0 gm/100 ml will result in a 0.8 mg/100 ml reduction in the total serum calcium concentration.

The measurement of bone density by photon absorption densitometry is a sensitive, noninvasive method, which can be used to detect and quantitate bone demineralization. This technique is considerably more sensitive than conventional radiographs, which require the loss of 30 to 40% of bone mineral before decreased mineralization can be identified with confidence.

Serum alkaline phosphatase can arise from bone, the liver, the gastrointestinal tract, and the placenta. Measurement of isoenzymes of alkaline phosphatase can be used to determine the origin. Heat fractionation is more widely used, but of more limited value. If the alkaline phosphatase is distinctly elevated and more than 80% heat-labile, bone origin is suspected.

DISORDERS OF MINERAL METABOLISM

SERUM CALCIUM The serum calcium concentration is normally maintained within a narrow range. Calcium levels reproducibly above or below this range require a diagnostic explanation. In contrast, the serum phosphate concentration normally varies more widely.

HYPERCALCEMIA Many patients with mild hypercalcemia, detected by routine chemical screening, are asymptomatic. Common symptoms attributable to moderate hypercalcemia include polyuria, constipation, anorexia, and nausea. With severe hypercalcemia, impaired mental function, stupor, and coma may supervene.

A reproducibly elevated total serum calcium concentration is rarely artifactual, although a minor increase in the serum calcium level, generally no more than 0.5 mg/100 ml, can be produced by prolonged tourniquet stasis prior to venipuncture. In at least one case, calcium binding to a serum paraprotein has been observed to cause elevation of the total serum calcium concentration without an elevation of the free calcium concentration. In most patients with paraproteinemia, however, the total serum calcium concentration is not elevated. Although the total serum calcium concentration may rise slightly after therapy with thiazide diuretics is initiated, this change is not maintained, and hypercalcemia in patients receiving chronic thiazide therapy should not be attributed to thiazide ingestion per se.

Causes of hypercalcemia are listed in Table 7-1. In the past, the diagnosis of primary hyperparathyroidism was essentially one of exclusion. The availability of PTH radioimmunoassays has made it possible to approach this diagnosis directly. Nonetheless, careful consideration of the diagnostic possibilities, and performance of the appropriate diagnostic studies, is in order. It should be recalled that multiple potential causes of hypercalcemia may be present in the same patient. For example, hypercalcemic patients with hyperparathyroidism and sarcoidosis, vitamin D intoxication and sarcoidosis, and thyrotoxicosis and multiple myeloma have been recognized.

Relatively mild hypercalcemia occurs in 10 to 20% of patients with thyrotoxicosis, especially in younger patients. Hypercalcemia is distinctly uncommon, and rarely severe, in patients with

Table 7-1
Differential diagnosis of hypercalcemia

A. Hyperparathyroidism

B. Malignant Disease
   1. Direct bone involvement–metastases to bone, multiple myeloma
   2. Indirect bone involvement–ectopic secretion of PTH, prostaglandins, or other humoral factors

C. Other
   1. Thyrotoxicosis
   2. Immobilization of patients with accelerated bone turnover (e.g., with Paget's disease)
   3. Vitamin D intoxication
   4. Vitamin A intoxication
   5. Milk-alkali syndrome
   6. Sarcoidosis
   7. Adrenocortical insufficiency

sarcoidosis. Such patients are inordinately sensitive to vitamin D. Thus, doses of vitamin D insufficient to cause hypercalcemia in normal subjects can produce major hypercalcemia in patients with sarcoidosis. Vitamin D intoxication can be diagnosed from the history and confirmed by measurement of the serum 25-OHD concentration. Similarly, hypercalcemia due to the chronic ingestion of large quantities of calcium along with absorbable alkali (the milk-alkali syndrome) can be strongly suspected from the history coupled with the findings of systemic alkalosis and azotemia. Although it was originally recognized in patients ingesting large quantities of milk and sodium bicarbonate, this syndrome can be produced by the excessive ingestion of calcium carbonate, a commonly used antacid. Mild hypercalcemia occurs in some patients with untreated Addison's disease. This may well be attributable to hemoconcentration. Accelerated calcium absorption from the gastrointestinal tract and diminished calcium excretion by the kidneys are theoretical possibilities, but studies in adrenalectomized animals do not support them. Hypercalcemia rarely occurs during immobilization of patients who do not have underlying bone disease and then it usually develops with virtually absolute immobilization (e.g., a full body cast). Patients with accelerated bone turnover, e.g., Paget's disease, commonly develop hypercalciuria and may develop hypercalcemia when put to bedrest.

In most hypercalcemic patients, the differential diagnosis can be rather easily narrowed to primary hyperparathyroidism* or hypercalcemia associated with malignant disease. Because of the effects of PTH on the kidneys, hypophosphatemia and a mild hyperchloremic acidosis are commonly present in patients with primary hyperparathyroidism. Indeed, a serum chloride to phosphate ratio of 33 or greater is highly suggestive of hyperparathyroidism. But, these findings are not invariably present and are not specific;

* Secondary hyperparathyroidism is not, by definition, associated with hypercalcemia. In certain unique situations in which the hypocalcemic stimulus is abruptly removed (e.g., renal transplantation), hypercalcemia may occur.

hypophosphatemia (less often hyperchloremia) is often a feature of the hypercalcemia of malignancy. Other indirect measurements, such as the determination of urinary cAMP excretion, may be of value, since cAMP excretion is lower in patients with hypercalcemia due to bone metastases than it is in patients with primary hyperparathyroidism. The distinction between patients with these disorders and normal subjects on the basis of cAMP excretion is not as clear cut.

In most patients, measurement of the serum PTH concentration clarifies this differential diagnosis. But, with most available PTH radioimmunoassays, a few patients with normal PTH levels and surgically proven primary hyperparathyroidism have been recognized. In the bulk of these cases, the serum PTH level, although within the normal range, is inappropriately high for the elevated serum calcium concentration. In an individual patient, however, this type of interpretation will result in a major decision based upon a subtle difference in the serum PTH concentration. Conversely, patients with hypercalcemia due to mechanisms other than primary hyperparathyroidism or the ectopic PTH syndrome have suppressed serum PTH levels that are often below the lower limit of assay sensitivity.

Furthermore, depending to a large extent upon the antiserum used, PTH-like molecules secreted from a nonparathyroid tumor (ectopic PTH syndrome) may cross-react.* Therefore, elevated PTH levels may be reported in some hypercalcemic patients who do not have primary hyperparathyroidism. Among the variety of tumors that have been associated with humoral hypercalcemia, the most common are carcinomas of the lung and genitourinary tract, particularly the kidneys. Therefore, in hypercalcemic patients without clinical evidence of neoplasm, normal chest films, intravenous urograms, and pelvic examinations constitute evidence against ectopic PTH secretion.

* Many patients with the ectopic PTH syndrome have lower levels of the biologically inactive, carboxy-terminal PTH fragment than patients with primary hyperparathyroidism. Thus, when an antiserum that recognizes the carboxy-terminal portion of the molecule is used, patients with the ectopic PTH syndrome are less likely to have elevated values.

The precise frequency of excessive secretion of PTH or a related molecule in patients with apparent humoral hypercalcemia is a matter of some debate. It seems clear, however, that some such patients have no evidence of excessive circulating PTH. Thus, other hypercalcemic substances, including prostaglandins of the E series, may be secreted by nonparathyroid tumors.

An uncommon but particularly difficult problem in differential diagnosis arises in hypercalcemic patients with a tumor that can cause humorally mediated hypercalcemia but that also is known to be associated with primary hyperparathyroidism. For example, hypercalcemia in patients with islet cell tumors of the pancreas is most often due to associated primary hyperparathyroidism. Recently, however, some patients with islet cell tumors and hypercalemia but without hyperparathyroidism have been recognized. Secretion of a hypercalcemic substance from the islet cell tumor is presumed to underlie the development of hypercalcemia. In such patients, measurement of PTH in samples obtained by venous catheterization of the small thyroidal veins that drain the parathyroid glands may be necessary. This procedure has also been utilized in the evaluation of patients with persistent hypercalcemia after previous parathyroid surgery. It should be emphasized that the small veins must be entered. Parathyroid hormone ratios as high as 2 : 1 between the large neck veins and the periphery have been seen in normocalcemic patients (and at least one hypercalcemic patient) without hyperparathyroidism.

The pathogenesis of primary hyperparathyroidism is unknown. Although its incidence is a matter of debate, parathyroid hyperplasia, rather than a solitary parathyroid adenoma, is found in many patients with primary hyperparathyroidism. Parathyroid carcinoma is a distinctly uncommon cause of primary hyperparathyroidism.

In many patients, the cause of hypercalcemia will be apparent after an initial history, physical examination, and routine laboratory studies. If this is not the case, the presence of hypercalcemia should be firmly established by repeated determinations of the total serum calcium concentration and measurement of the free serum calcium concentration and a search for the hypercalcemic mechanism that begins with measurement of the serum PTH and serum thyroxine, performance of immunoelectrophoresis on serum, urine, or both, and radiographic examination of the chest and urinary tract. If metastatic disease is suspected, the appropriate bone films, bone scans, or both are in order. If these studies do not disclose the origin of the hypercalcemia, specific studies of cortisol secretion and serum 25-OHD levels can be performed. Idiopathic hypercalcemia is not a tenable diagnosis in adult patients.

Once a diagnosis of primary hyperparathyroidism is made, the possibility of a multiple endocrine neoplasia syndrome should be considered. These are of at least two types. Multiple endocrine neoplasia, type 1, includes (a) pituitary tumors, which are often functional, i.e., they hypersecrete growth hormone, prolactin, or both (b) primary hyperparathyroidism, and (c) islet cell tumors of the pancreas, which most often secrete insulin or gastrin, but may secrete a variety of hormones. Multiple endocrine neoplasia, type 2, includes (a) medullary carcinoma of the thyroid with hypersecretion of calcitonin, (b) primary hyperparathyroidism, and (c) pheochromocytoma.

HYPOCALCEMIA Major hypocalcemia causes tetany. Tetany may be overt with paresthesias, muscle cramps, and carpopedal spasm. Laryngeal spasm and seizures are rare manifestations of hypocalcemia in adult patients. Acute hypocalcemia is more likely to be symptomatic than is chronic hypocalcemia of similar magnitude. Patients with latent tetany have no symptoms (or nonspecific symptoms), although signs of hypocalcemia can be elicited. Chvostek's sigh (twitching of the facial muscles, particularly at the angle of the mouth, with tapping over the facial nerve anterior to the ear) is commonly present in hypocalcemic patients, but may also be seen in approximately 10% of adult patients in the absence of hypocalcemia. Trousseau's sign (carpopedal spasm during occlusion of arterial flow in the upper extremity) is more specific for hypocalcemia.* Occlusion should be maintained for 3

* Trousseau's sign has been reported in normocalcemic patients with the thoracic outlet syndrome, and the author has seen it in a normocalcemic patient with the carpal tunnel syndrome.

minutes in the absence of carpopedal spasm before it is concluded that Trousseau's sign is absent.

Clinical tetany is not specific for hypocalcemia. Tetany may be produced by systemic alkalosis, presumably due to alterations in membrane excitability as a direct effect of elevated pH rather than to a decrease in the free calcium concentration. This may be due to either metabolic or respiratory alkalosis. Indeed, the acute respiratory alkalosis of the hyperventilation syndrome may be the most common cause of tetany. Tetany may also occur in magnesium-depleted patients.

In contrast to elevation of the total serum calcium concentration, depression of the total serum calcium concentration is often of little clinical significance in that it is due to hypoproteinemia with a resulting decrease in the protein-bound calcium fraction. In such instances, the free serum calcium concentration is normal. A small artifactual decrease in the serum calcium concentration may occur if separation of the serum from the formed elements of the blood is delayed.

In general, true hypocalcemia develops when PTH, or vitamin D, is deficient or when there is an abnormality in the metabolism of PTH or vitamin D or their biologic effectiveness is decreased. Patients in chronic negative calcium balance, due to low dietary calcium, calcium malabsorption, hypercalciuria, etc., generally do not develop hypocalcemia because of a compensatory increase in PTH secretion [and, perhaps, an increase in 1,25-$(OH)_2D$ formation], although osteopenia may develop (see below). Exceptions to this generalization would include patients in whom there is an acute, intensive hypocalcemic stimulus, such as acute hyperphosphatemia and, perhaps, acute pancreatitis. Symptomatic hypocalcemia does occur in the latter disorders, perhaps because the compensatory mechanisms are at least temporarily overwhelmed. Chronic renal failure is a common cause of hypocalcemia. At least two mechanisms are involved: (a) phosphate retention with hyperphosphatemia and reciprocal hypocalcemia and (b) vitamin D resistance, perhaps due to decreased renal production of 1,25-$(OH)_2D$.

Hypoparathyroidism is most often secondary to thyroid or

parathyroid surgery. Patients with idiopathic hypoparathyroidism are almost invariably detected in infancy or childhood. Idiopathic hypoparathyroidism may be associated with other hormonal deficiencies, notably primary adrenocortical insufficiency, primary hypogonadism, and diabetes mellitus. Only rarely have patients with acquired, nonsurgical hypoparathyroidism due to chronic iron overload, massive doses of ^{131}I for thyroid carcinoma, or metastases to the parathyroid glands been reported. Recently, an increasing number of patients with symptomatic hypocalcemia and magnesium depletion have been recognized. Hypocalcemia in such patients does not respond to calcium supplementation but does respond dramatically to magnesium replenishment. Although the mechanisms are not entirely clear, impaired PTH secretion would appear to play a role in the pathogenesis of hypomagnesemic hypocalcemia.

Pseudohypoparathyroidism is a rare, often familial disorder characterized by hypocalcemia and hyperphosphatemia indistinguishable from those seen in hypoparathyroidism. In contrast to hypoparathyroidism, however, patients with pseudohypoparathyroidism often exhibit a characteristic phenotype (including short stature, brachydactyly, short neck, round face, and subcutaneous calcification); these patients also have elevated serum PTH levels. Infused parathyroid hormone does not produce the normal increase in urinary cAMP or phosphate excretion in such patients, suggesting that resistance to the biologic effects of PTH underlies the development of hypocalcemia in pseudohypoparathyroidism. Patients who exhibit a similar phenotype but who do not have hypocalcemia ("pseudopseudohypoparathyroidism") have been recognized; whether they represent a distinct entity or a part of the spectrum of pseudohypoparathyroidism remains to be established.

Dietary vitamin D deficiency is distinctly rare in this country. In a variety of disorders, however, abnormalities in the metabolism of vitamin D are either suspected or proven to occur. For example, serum 25-OHD levels have been shown to be low in patients with chronic liver disease (biliary cirrhosis) and in patients treated with drugs (diphenylhydantoin, phenobarbital) that induce hepatic enzymes, and serum 1,25-$(OH)_2D$ levels have been found to be low in patients with chronic renal disease. Although hypocalcemia may occur in vitamin D deficient or resistant states, hypophosphatemia is the more consistent, and generally the more striking, finding.

Hypocalcemia is not a feature of the hypercalcitoninemic syndrome associated with medullary carcinoma of the thyroid.

In summary, a reproducibly decreased total serum calcium concentration should prompt examination of the serum protein levels. If the latter are depressed, the presence of true hypocalcemia can be confirmed or ruled out by measurement of the free calcium concentration. When the etiology of hypocalcemia is not readily apparent, the serum PTH level should be measured, especially in patients with hyperphosphatemia. Although most available PTH assays are insufficiently sensitive to distinguish low from normal PTH levels, it is generally assumed that a PTH level that is not elevated in the presence of a low free calcium concentration indicates inadequate PTH secretion. Serum and urinary magnesium should be measured routinely in patients with unexplained hypocalcemia. The study of hypocalcemic disorders and the clinical evaluation of hypocalcemic patients will be facilitated by the greater availability of serum 25-OHD and 1,25-$(OH)_2D$ determinations.

SERUM MAGNESIUM Magnesium metabolism and its role in the pathogenesis of human disease are incompletely understood. It has been emphasized that, at least in some circumstances, there is little correlation between the serum and tissue magnesium levels. In patients with kwashiorkor, for example, depletion of muscle magnesium may coincide with normal serum magnesium concentrations, whereas during experimental magnesium depletion, erythrocyte magnesium levels fall only slightly despite the development of hypomagnesemia and striking hypomagnesiuria. Nonetheless, serum and urine are the only readily available fluids for clinical evaluation of magnesium status.

HYPERMAGNESEMIA Severe hypermagnesemia has been associated with neuromuscular depression, atrioventricular block, and depression of the central nervous system. Although hypermagnesemia may occur in patients with adrenocortical insufficiency and during the ingestion of large quantities of magnesium (especially in cathartics), clinically significant hypermagnesemia is virtually limited to patients with renal failure who also have a generous magnesium intake.

HYPOMAGNESEMIA Experimental magnesium depletion in man produces a clinical syndrome characterized by irritability, apathy, weakness, anorexia, and nausea, often with evidence of tetany including a Trousseau's sign. In addition, seizures and coma have been attributed to magnesium depletion.

Various causes of magnesium depletion are outlined in Table 7-2. Clinically significant hypomagnesemia is most often seen in

Table 7-2
Recognized causes of magnesium depletion

A. Inadequate Intake

B. Malabsorption

C. Excessive Losses
- 1. Renal
  - a. Alcoholism[a]
  - b. Hyperparathyroidism[b]
  - c. Hyperthyroidism
  - d. Hyperaldosteronism
  - e. Diuretic therapy
  - f. Syndrome of inappropriate ADH secretion
  - g. Diabetic ketoacidosis
  - h. Idiopathic
- 2. Extrarenal
  - a. Lactation
  - b. Prolonged loss of body fluids

[a] Deficient dietary magnesium may well contribute.
[b] Hypomagnesemia may become apparent after parathyroidectomy.

patients with chronic malabsorption (including patients who have undergone intestinal bypass surgery for obesity) or chronic alcoholism.

In summary, the serum and urine magnesium should be measured in patients with any of the nonspecific symptoms listed above and a clinical state known to be associated with magnesium depletion, particularly in the presence of unexplained hypocalcemia.

OSTEOPENIA This is a general term used to describe diminished bone density. It embraces the traditional categories of metabolic bone disease–osteoporosis, osteomalacia (rickets), and osteitis fibrosa. The following classification is clinically useful:

Osteoporosis–Osteopenia with diminished bone mass but histologically normal bone.
Osteomalacia–Osteopenia with defective calcification of osteoid.
Osteitis fibrosa–Osteopenia with increased osteoclastic activity.

Osteoporosis is manifested clinically by fractures that often involve the vertebrae. The serum calcium, phosphorus, and alkaline phosphatase concentrations are typically normal. Bone pain and deformity, as well as fractures, occur in patients with *osteomalacia*. Typically, the serum alkaline phosphatase is elevated and the serum phosphorus depressed. The serum calcium concentration may be normal or somewhat low. Radiographically, pseudofractures (straight radiolucent bands with increased radiodensity along either side) are classic, although often absent findings in osteomalacia. Patients with *osteitis fibrosa* most often exhibit only osteopenia radiographically, although subperiosteal resorption and cystic bone changes may occur. Circulating PTH or PTH-like substances should be elevated in patients with osteitis fibrosa.

Various disorders associated with osteoporosis, osteomalacia, and osteitis fibrosa are listed in Table 7-3. It should be emphasized that although plain radiographs and bone densitometry serve to document the presence of osteopenia and, to some extent, quantitate its degree, these techniques do not usually distinguish

Table 7-3
Disorders associated with various forms of osteopenia

A. Osteoporosis
1. Osteoporosis of unknown etiology ("postmenopausal" or "senile" osteoporosis)
2. Endocrinologic disorders
    a. Thyrotoxicosis
    b. Cushing's syndrome (including the iatrogenic form)
    c. Hyperparathyroidism
    d. Turner's and Klinefelter's syndromes
3. Metabolic disorders
    a. Diabetes mellitus
    b. Osteogenesis imperfecta
    c. Hypophosphatasia
    d. Others–Homocystinuria, Marfan's syndrome, Ehlers-Danlos syndrome, Riley-Day syndrome, copper deficiency
4. Immobilization
5. Juvenile osteoporosis (prepubertal, transient)
6. Miscellaneous
    a. Chronic calcium deficiency
    b. Chronic liver disease, alcoholism
    c. Malignant disorders–multiple myeloma, leukemia, macroglobulinemia
    d. Heparin excess (? the mechanism of osteoporosis in systemic mastocytosis)
    e. Others–Down's syndrome, cystic fibrosis

B. Osteomalacia (and Rickets)
1. Dietary vitamin D deficiency
    a. Absolute
    b. Relative–associated with accelerated vitamin D metabolism (e.g., therapy with diphenylhydantoin, phenobarbital, or both; ? aging)
2. Intestinal disorders
    a. Intestinal or pancreatic disease with malabsorption
    b. Gastrectomy
    c. Chronic liver disease–especially biliary cirrhosis
3. Renal disorders
    a. Chronic renal failure
    b. Renal tubular acidosis
    c. Familial hypophosphatemia (including vitamin D resistant rickets)

        d. Vitamin D dependency
    4. Miscellaneous
        a. Chronic phosphate depletion
        b. Tumor-associated (especially skin or bone tumors)
        c. Iatrogenic–diphenylhydantoin, phenobarbital, fluoride, diphosphonates
        d. Associated with osteopetrosis

C. Osteitis Fibrosa
    1. Primary hyperparathyroidism (and ectopic secretion of PTH-like factors)
    2. Secondary hyperparthyroidism
        a. Deficient calcium intake or absorption
        b. Excessive calcium loss
        c. Phosphate retention (e.g., chronic renal failure)
        d. Vitamin D disorders
    3. Pseudohypoparathyroidism (renal, but not bone, resistance to PTH)

---

among the three major categories of osteopenia. When the mechanism of osteopenia is not apparent after the basic studies have been performed, and osteopenia is a clinically significant finding, bone biopsy is indicated. Semiquantitative study of undecalcified bone, which can be obtained from the iliac crest under local anesthesia, permits accurate classification of the bone disease and rational therapy. The administration of tetracycline several days before biopsy results in fluorescent labeling of the calcification front, thus permitting accurate definition of osteomalacia (increased osteoid with diminished to absent calcification fronts) if present.

Paget's disease of bone (osteitis deformans) is a common, but often asymptomatic disorder characterized by rapid bone turnover. A striking elevation of serum alkaline phosphatase of bone origin and typical radiographic findings, most often in the pelvis and femur, are characteristic. The serum calcium, phosphate, magnesium, PTH, and 25-OHD are normal. In severe cases, bone pain and deformity, especially of the lower extremities, and enlargement of the skull, with compression of nerves passing through cranial foramina (auditory, optic, etc.), may occur. Major hypercalciuria, and occasionally hypercalcemia, may occur when patients with Paget's disease are immobilized.

UROLITHIASIS Recognized causes of urinary tract calculi are outlined in Table 7-4. After thorough evaluation, the mechanism of stone formation will remain unclear in approximately 25% of patients with recurrent urinary tract calculi. Nonetheless, the availability of effective therapy for several of the recognized causes of stone formation makes diagnostic evaluation of all patients with recurrent calculi mandatory.

Most patients with recurrent, radiopaque urinary tract calculi exhibit hypercalciuria. The widely used upper limits of normal for urinary calcium excretion on an unrestricted diet (300 mg/24

Table 7-4
Differential diagnosis of urolithiasis

A. Hypercalciuric States
   1. With hypercalcemia (see Table 7-1)
   2. Without hypercalcemia
      a. Idiopathic hypercalciuria
      b. Renal tubular acidosis (distal type)
      c. Accelerated bone turnover (e.g., Paget's disease) especially with immobilization

B. Uric Acid Calculi (with or without hyperuricemia)

C. Magnesium Ammonium Phosphate Calculi—Urinary Tract Infection

D. Other
   1. Cystinuria
   2. Renal tubular acidosis
   3. Hyperoxaluria
   4. ? Hypomagnesiuria

E. Idiopathic

hours in adult men and 250 mg/24 hours in adult women) are conservative. Although patients in whom these values are exceeded certainly have hypercalciuria, one cannot be certain that patients in whom calcium excretion approaches these values do not have hypercalciuria. Some have advocated reevaluation of patients who excrete more than 175 mg of calcium/24 hours by placing them on a low calcium (200 mg) diet for 3 to 4 days, since calcium excretion should fall to less than 150 mg/24 hours in normal subjects on such a diet. A minority of hypercalciuric stone-formers will be found to have hypercalcemia, and the differential diagnosis becomes that of hypercalcemia. The bulk of hypercalciuric stone-formers do not have hypercalcemia. Some of them will be found to have recognized causes of accelerated bone turnover (e.g., Paget's disease) or of decreased renal calcium reabsorption (renal tubular acidosis), although most will not. Patients with hypercalciuria, normocalcemia, and no recognized bone or renal disease are classified as having idiopathic hypercalciuria, the most common cause of urinary tract calculi in men. For unexplained reasons, this disorder rarely occurs in women. Whether idiopathic hypercalciuria represents a primary renal defect in calcium reabsorption or a primary gastrointestinal hyperabsorption of calcium is a matter of debate. It is likely that different mechanisms are operative in different patients. Secondary hyperparathyroidism (consistent with the renal calcium leak hypothesis) has been described in patients with idiopathic hypercalciuria by some investigators but questioned by others. Mild to moderate hypophosphatemia (also consistent with the renal calcium leak hypothesis) occurs not infrequently in patients with idiopathic hypercalciuria. Elevated serum 1,25-$(OH)_2D$ levels in such patients have been reported.

Other relatively common urinary tract calculi are uric acid stones and magnesium ammonium phosphate stones. Uric acid calculi may occur in the presence or absence of hyperuricemia. In contrast to calcium containing calculi, uric acid calculi are typically radiolucent. One mechanism for the formation of uric acid stones in the absence of hyperuricosuria is the persistent excretion of urine with an inappropriately low pH. Uric acid is least soluble at low pH levels. In contrast, magnesium ammonium phosphate calculi most often occur in urine made alkaline by urinary tract infection with urea-splitting microorganisms. This poses a difficult therapeutic problem, since the presence of calculi favors continued infection and continued infection favors continued stone formation.

Relatively uncommon causes of urinary tract calculi include cystinuria, renal tubular acidosis, hyperoxaluria, and perhaps, hypomagnesiuria. Although hexagonal cystine crystals can often be seen in acidified urine of cystinuric patients, this finding is not diagnostic and qualitative or quantitative urinary cystine determinations are preferable. The form of renal tubular acidosis commonly associated with urolithiasis, nephrocalcinosis, or both is characterized by an inability to acidify the urine to a pH of less than 5.5 under any conditions and is usually associated with overt systemic hyperchloremic acidosis. Hyperoxaluria occurs rarely as a primary metabolic disorder; urinary stone formation and progressive nephron destruction are the rule. Recently, several varieties of acquired hyperoxaluria with stone formation have been recognized, most notably that following distal ileal resection or bypass. Other causes of acquired hyperoxaluria include high dietary oxalate intake (e.g., rhubarb, tea), pyridoxine deficiency, ethylene glycol ingestion, and methoxyflurane anesthesia. It has been observed that patients with unexplained calcium oxalate stone formation often have a urine magnesium to calcium ratio of less than 0.5, and it has been suggested that relative hypomagnesiuria may contribute to stone formation.

In summary, patients with recurrent urinary tract calculi should have repeated measurements of the serum calcium, phosphorus, alkaline phosphatase, and uric acid levels and of the urinary excretion of calcium and uric acid, as well as routine examination and culture of the urine. Every effort, including straining of the urine, should be made to obtain calculi for chemical analysis, and the collecting system should be visualized by intravenous urography. If hypercalcemia is detected, the appropriate diagnostic evaluation described earlier should be carried out. If the mechanism of stone formation is not readily apparent, measurements of urinary cystine and oxalate are in order, and the serum electrolyte and arterial and urine pH should be examined.

CALCITONIN As yet, clinical syndromes directly attributable to calcitonin excess or deficit have not been clearly defined. An elevated plasma calcitonin level has, however, been shown to be a useful marker for medullary carcinoma of the thyroid. Indeed, in studies of relatives of patients with medullary carcinomas of the thyroid, a sharp increase in the plasma calcitonin concentration during an infusion of calcium (15 mg/kg over 4 hours) has led to the discovery of medullary carcinomas even in the absence of clinical evidence of thyroid disease and of elevated basal calcitonin levels.

Elevated plasma calcitonin levels alone cannot be considered to be diagnostic of medullary carcinoma of the thyroid. Elevated calcitonin levels have been noted in several patients with common malignancies (e.g., carcinoma of the lung or breast) and in patients with a variety of less common neoplastic disorders, including carcinoid tumors, malignant melanomas, and islet cell tumors of the pancreas.

SUGGESTED READING

1. Avioli LV, Krane SM (eds): Metabolic Bone Disease, Volume 1. Academic Press, New York, 1977.
2. Avioli LV, Krane SM (eds): Metabolic Bone Disease, Volume 2. Academic Press, New York, In Press.
3. Ladenson JH, Lewis JW, Boyd JC: Failure of total calcium corrected for protein, albumin and pH to correctly assess free calcium status. *J Clin Endocrinol Metab* 46:986, 1978.
4. Flueck JA, DiBella FP, Edis AJ, Kehrwald JM, Arnaud CD: Immunoheterogeneity of parathyroid hormone in venous effluent serum from hyperfunctioning parathyroid glands. *J Clin Invest* 60:1367, 1977.
5. Heath H, Sizemore GW: Plasma calcitonin in normal man. Differences between men and women. *J Clin Invest* 60:1135, 1977.

6. Parthemore JG, Deftos LJ: Calcitonin secretion in normal human subjects. *J Clin Endocrinol Metab* 47:184, 1978.
7. Schneider AB, Sherwood LM: Calcium homeostasis and the pathogenesis and management of hypercalcemic disorders. *Metabolism* 23:975, 1974.
8. Mallette LE, Bilezikian JB, Heath DA, Aurbach GD: Primary hyperparathyroidism: Clinical and biochemical features. *Medicine* 53:127, 1974.
9. Broadus AE, Deftos LJ, Bartter FC: Effects of the intravenous administration of calcium on nephrogenous cyclic AMP. *J Clin Endocrinol Metab* 46:477, 1978.
10. Benson RC Jr, Riggs BL, Pickard BM, Arnaud CD: Radioimmunoassay of parathyroid hormone in hypercalcemic patients with malignant disease. *Amer J Med* 56:821, 1974.
11. Seyberth HW, Segre GV, Morgan JL, Sweetman BJ, Potts JT, Oates JA: Prostaglandins as mediators of hypercalcemic associated with certain types of cancer. *N Engl J Med* 293:1278, 1975.
12. Burman KD, Monchik JM, Earll JM, Wartofsky L: Ionized and total serum calcium and parathyroid hormone in hyperthyroidism. *Ann Intern Med* 84:668, 1976.
13. Wiberg JJ, Turner GG, Nuttall FQ: Effect of phosphate or magnesium cathartics on serum calcium. *Arch Intern Med* 138:1114, 1978.
14. Freitag J, Martin KJ, Hruska KA, Anderson C, Conrades M, Ladenson J, Klahr S, Slatopolsky E: Impaired parathyroid hormone metabolism in patients with chronic renal failure. *N Engl J Med* 298:29, 1978.
15. Anast CS, Winnacker J, Forte LR, Burns TW: Impaired release of parathyroid hormone in magnesium deficiency. *J Clin Endocrinol Metab* 42:707, 1976.
16. Marx SJ, Aurbach GD: Heterogeneous hormonal disorder in pseudohypoparathyroidism. *N Engl J Med* 296:169, 1977.
17. Shils ME: Experimental human magnesium depletion. *Medicine* 48:61, 1969.
18. Hausler MR, McCain TA: Basic and clinical concepts related to vitamin D metabolism and action. *N Engl J Med* 297:974 and 1041, 1977.
19. Avioli LV (ed): Vitamin D metabolites: Their clinical importance. *Arch Intern Med* 138:835, 1978.
20. Recker RR, Saville PD, Heaney RP: Effect of estrogens and calcium carbonate on bone loss in postmenopausal women. *Ann Intern Med* 87:649, 1977.
21. Hahn TJ, Hendin BA, Scharp CH et al: Serum 25-hydroxycalcif-

erol levels and bone mass in children on chronic anticonvulsant therapy. *N Engl J Med* 292:550, 1975.

22. Yendt ET: Renal calculi. *Can Med Assoc J* 102:479, 1970.
23. Bordier P, Ryckewart A, Gueris J, Rasmussen H: On the pathogenesis of so-called idiopathic hypercalciuria. *Amer J Med* 63:398, 1977.
24. Caldas AE, Gray RW, Lemann J Jr: The simultaneous measurement of vitamin D metabolites in plasma. Studies in healthy adults and in patients with calcium nephrolithiasis. *J Lab Clin Med* 91:840, 1978.
25. Coe FL: Treated and untreated recurrent calcium nephrolithiasis in patients with idiopathic hypercalciuria, hyperuricosuria or no metabolic disorder. *Ann Intern Med* 87:404, 1977.
26. Pak CYC, Fetner C, Townsend J, Brinkley L, Northcutt C, Barilla DE, Kadesky M, Peters P: Evaluation of calcium urolithiasis in ambulatory patients. Comparison of results with those of inpatient evaluation. *Amer J Med* 64:979, 1978.

8

THE HYPERLIPOPROTEINEMIAS

Hyperlipoproteinemia is a common biochemical finding often associated with arteriosclerotic vascular disease and at times presenting with clinical manifestations directly attributable to the elevated lipid levels. The premise, which remains to be proven, that therapeutic reduction of elevated lipoprotein levels will retard the development of arteriosclerotic vascular disease has stimulated clinical interest in this group of disorders.

Of the circulating lipids, major emphasis has been placed on the cholesterol and triglyceride concentrations. The term *hyperlipidemia* refers to elevation of the level of one or both of these lipids. But, lipids circulate in plasma in water-soluble complexes with specific proteins (apoproteins); these complexes are the lipoproteins, and elevation of a given lipoprotein class is termed *hyperlipoproteinemia*. There are four major lipoprotein classes:

1. Chylomicrons, containing mostly triglycerides of dietary origin and only small quantities of cholesterol.
2. Very low density lipoproteins (VLDL), containing mostly endogenously synthesized triglycerides and only 5 to 10% of the circulating cholesterol.
3. Low density lipoproteins (LDL), containing 50 to 75% of the

circulating cholesterol and relatively small quantities of triglycerides.

4. High density lipoproteins (HDL), containing 25 to 40% of the circulating cholesterol and relatively small quantities of triglycerides.

It is currently believed that the LDL are formed from VLDL via intermediates sometimes termed the intermediate density lipoproteins (IDL). A simplified view of triglyceride and cholesterol transport is illustrated in Fig. 8-1.

Hyperlipoproteinemia can be primary or secondary to another disorder. Primary hyperlipoproteinemia can often be shown to be familial. Five types of familial hyperlipoproteinemia are listed in

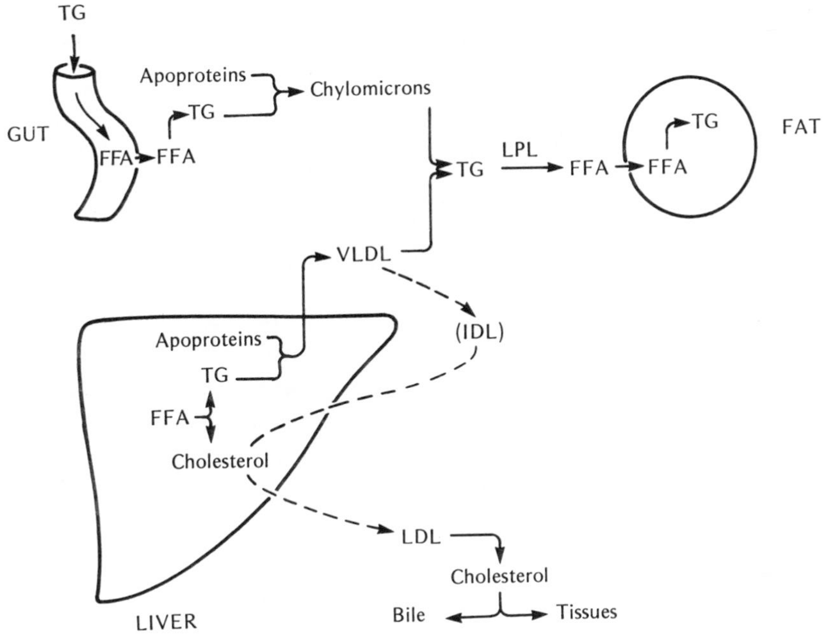

FIG. 8-1. Overview of cholesterol and triglyceride (TG) transport; FFA, free fatty acids; LPL, lipoprotein lipase; VLDL, very low density lipoproteins; LDL, low density lipoproteins; IDL, intermediate density lipoproteins.

Table 8-1
Familial types of hyperlipoproteinemias (Frederickson and Levy)

I. Familial Lipoprotein Lipase-Deficient Hyperchylomicronemia
II. Familial Hyperbetalipoproteinemia
III. Familial "Broad Beta" Disease
IV. Familial Hyperprebetalipoproteinemia
V. Familial Hyperprebetalipoproteinemia and Hyperchylomicronemia

Table 8-1. This classification, proposed by Frederickson and Levy, will be used as the basis of the discussion of hyperlipoproteinemia that follows. A more recently recognized familial hyperlipoproteinemia, combined hyperlipoproteinemia, will also be discussed.

Although the role of elevated lipoprotein levels as a risk factor for arteriosclerotic vascular disease has been traditionally emphasized, an apparently protective effect of HDL (and HDL-cholesterol) has recently been recognized. Thus, persons with higher levels of HDL-cholesterol appear to have lesser degrees of arteriosclerosis.

ANALYTICAL METHODS

A great deal can be deduced from simple observation of 18- to 24-hour refrigerated plasma obtained from a patient in the fasting state. Turbidity of the plasma indicates a major increase in the triglyceride concentration. A thick layer of "cream" floating at the top of the plasma indicates the presence of circulating chylomicrons.*

The next step in the evaluation of patients with hyperlipoproteinemia is the measurement of the fasting serum cholesterol and triglyceride concentrations. Samples should be obtained after a minimal fast of 12 hours and at a time when the patient has been

* The appearance of refrigerated plasma from normal and hyperlipoproteinemic patients has been nicely illustrated. (Murphy BF: Management of hyperlipidemias. *J Amer Med Assoc* 230:1683, 1974.)

ingesting his usual diet for at least 2 weeks. Negative caloric balance (weight loss) will result in a lowering of the cholesterol and triglyceride levels. Furthermore, major deviations in dietary composition from the norm can result in an elevation of certain lipoprotein classes. For example, ingestion of a very high carbohydrate diet by a normal subject results in elevation of VLDL and, therefore, of triglyceride levels (carbohydrate induction), often above the upper limits of normal. Alcohol ingestion has a similar effect. It should be recalled that "normal" levels are determined from subjects ingesting a "normal" diet. Fasting cholesterol and triglyceride levels should, in general, be measured on several occasions in view of their variability.

Ideally, normal serum cholesterol and triglyceride concentrations should be determined in a given locality by the methods used in the local laboratory. Since there is a distinct increase in the cholesterol concentration, and a significant increase in the triglyceride concentration, with increasing age in the normal American population, age-adjusted normal values are frequently used. It should be emphasized that normal ranges are statistically derived and that a single measurement of cholesterol or triglycerides that exceeds the normal range does not establish the presence of hyperlipidemia. Indeed, if 90% limits of the normal population are used to define the normal range, 5% of normal subjects sampled will be expected to have values above "normal." Again, particularly in the patient with marginally elevated values, repeated measurements of the fasting cholesterol and triglyceride levels are in order.

Although uncommon, it is possible for a patient to have hyperlipoproteinemia in the absence of hyperlipidemia. For example, a patient with elevated LDL (and, therefore, elevated LDL cholesterol) could have a normal total serum cholesterol if there were an associated decrease in HDL (and HDL cholesterol).

The presence of hyperlipoproteinemia can be conclusively established and defined by quantitative determination of lipoprotein levels by ultracentrifugation. It is impractical, however, to employ ultracentrifugation for all patients screened for hyperlipoprotein-

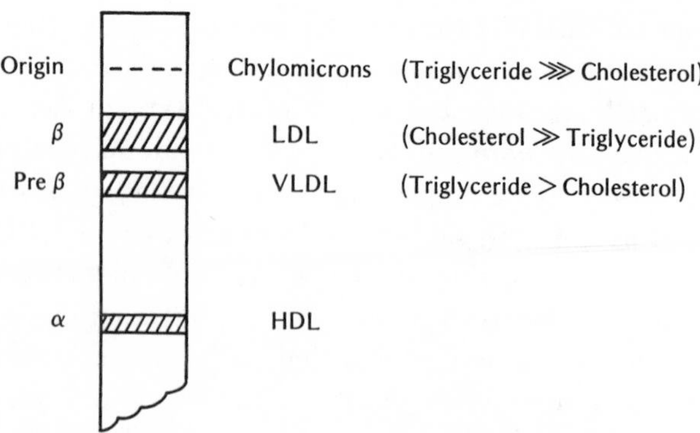

FIG 8-2. Diagram of the normal lipoprotein electrophoresis on paper. The designations of the bands and the corresponding lipoprotein classes are indicated.

emia or even all patients with established hyperlipidemia. In recent years it has become popular to perform lipoprotein electrophoresis on the serum of fasting patients with hyperlipidemia as an adjunct in classifying their hyperlipoproteinemia. Qualitative serum lipoprotein electrophoresis is now widely available and relatively inexpensive, although the merits of its routine use have been seriously questioned, as will be discussed later in this chapter. Paper electrophoresis is perhaps most widely used. As illustrated in Fig. 8-2, on paper electrophoresis chylomicrons remain at the origin, LDL occupy the beta band, VLDL occupy the pre-beta band, and HDL occupy the alpha band.

THE HYPERLIPOPROTEINEMIAS

The biochemical findings, and definitions, of the five types of hyperlipoproteinemia are outlined in Table 8-2. The clinical features of the hyperlipoproteinemias are outlined in Table 8-3.

In general, once the presence of hyperlipoproteinemia is established, and the type determined, possible secondary causes are sought. In the absence of secondary causes (phenocopies), the hyperlipoproteinemia is assumed to be primary. Although the fa-

Table 8-2

Laboratory features of familial hyperlipoproteinemias

TYPE	ABNORMALITY	APPEARANCE OF PLASMA	CHOLESTEROL	TRIGLYCERIDES	C/T[a] RATIO	PAPER ELECTROPHORESIS	OTHER[b]
I	Increased chylomicrons	Cream/clear	Increased	Increased	<0.2	Band at origin	
II	Increased LDL						
IIa	With normal VLDL	Clear	Increased	Normal	–	Increased β band	
IIb	With increased VLDL	Clear (or turbid)	Increased	Increased	>1.5	Increased β+ increased pre-β bands	
III	Increased VLDL of abnormal composition (IDL)	Faint cream/turbid	Increased	Increased	~1.0	Increased β band (broad β)	VLDL cholesterol : triglyceride >0.3, floating β (β-VLDL) on UC
IV	Increased VLDL	Turbid	Increased or Normal	Increased	–	Increased pre-β band	
V	Increased chylomicrons + VLDL	Cream/turbid	Increased	Increased	0.15–0.6	Band at origin + increased pre-β band	

[a] C/T ratio, cholesterol : triglyceride ratio.
[b] UC, ultracentrifugation.

Table 8-3
Clinical features of familial hyperlipoproteinemias

TYPE	INHERITANCE	RELATIVE FREQUENCY	XANTHOMAS	PREMATURE VASCULAR DISEASE	ABNORMAL GLUCOSE TOLERANCE
I	Autosomal recessive	Least common	Eruptive	No	No
II	Autosomal dominant	Common	Tendon, Tuberous (Planar-homozygotes)	Yes	No
III	Autosomal recessive	Uncommon	Planar (Tuberous)	Yes	Yes
IV	Autosomal dominant	Common	(Eruptive)	Yes	Yes
V	? Autosomal dominant	Uncommon	Eruptive	?	Yes

OTHER CLINICAL FEATURES		PHENOCOPIES	
Episodic abdominal pain, hepatomegaly common, onset in childhood	TYPE I:	Diabetes Hypothyroidism Dysglobulinemias (especially systemic lupus erythematosus)	Pancreatitis Oral contraceptives Glucocorticoids
Abnormal lipids from birth, heterozygotes—II or tendon xanthomas, in 1st degree relative homozygotes—LDL twice heterozygotes or II in both parents	TYPE II:	Hypothyroidism Biliary obstruction Dysglobulinemias	Nephrotic syndrome Porphyria
Rarely detected before age 20, often dramatic response to therapy	TYPE III:	Diabetes Hypothyroidism Dysglobulinemias	
Expression generally delayed until adulthood	TYPES IV AND V:	Diabetes Hypothyroidism Alcoholism Pancreatitis Renal failure	Nephrotic syndrome Dysglobulinemias Oral contraceptives Glucocorticoids
Expression generally delayed until adulthood, may have episodic abdominal pain and hepatomegaly			

milial nature of a primary hyperlipoproteinemia can often be strongly suspected from the family history, a study of family members is required to prove this point.

Abnormal lipid deposits, *xanthomas*, are important clinical findings in patients with hyperlipoproteinemia. Although xanthelasma and arcus corneae commonly occur in the absence of hyperlipoproteinemia, and rare patients with tendon xanthomas and normal lipoprotein levels have been described, subcutaneous (tuberous) xanthomas, flat, orange-colored (planar) xanthomas, and yellow, red-based (eruptive) xanthomas are virtually pathognomonic of hyperlipoproteinemia.

TYPE I HYPERLIPOPROTEINEMIA The presence of chylomicrons and the absence of increased VLDL in fasting plasma characterize the type I abnormality. A layer of "cream" (chylomicrons) is present at the top of 18- to 24-hour refrigerated plasma; the remainder of the plasma is clear. Major elevation of triglyceride levels, with a cholesterol to triglyceride ratio of less than 0.2, is characteristic. The only abnormal finding on paper electrophoresis is a band at the origin (chylomicrons).

Type I hyperlipoproteinemia results from failure to clear chylomicrons derived from dietary fat due to a deficiency of the enzyme lipoprotein lipase. The chylomicrons disappear over several days when fat is removed from the diet. This relatively rare type of hyperlipoproteinemia usually becomes clinically apparent in childhood with episodes of abdominal pain and eruptive xanthomas and with progressive hepatosplenomegaly.

TYPE II HYPERLIPOPROTEINEMIA Elevated LDL concentrations characterize the type II abnormality, which is one of the most common forms of hyperlipoproteinemia. It has been subdivided as follows:

IIa. Clear refrigerated plasma, elevated cholesterol, but normal triglyceride concentrations, and an increased beta band on lipoprotein electrophoresis.

IIb. Clear (or turbid) refrigerated plasma, elevated cholesterol *and* triglyceride concentrations (with a cholesterol to triglyceride ratio of greater than 1.5), and increased beta and pre-beta bands on lipoprotein electrophoresis.

Type II hyperlipoproteinemia is an autosomal dominant disorder strongly associated with premature arteriosclerotic vascular disease. Tendon and tuberous xanthomas occur rather commonly; planar xanthomas occur in the rare homozygotes.

In a series of elegant studies, Brown and Goldstein have greatly clarified the molecular mechanisms of the hypercholesterolemia typical of type II hyperlipoproteinemia. Normally, LDL interact with cell surface receptors with subsequent cellular internalization of LDL, degradation of the protein component by lysosomal enzymes, and liberation of free cholesterol, which suppresses cellular cholesterol synthesis and is utilized as a source of cholesterol by the cell. Thus, this system provides a mechanism for cholesterol clearance from the plasma by cells with suppression of cholesterol synthesis in those cells. Studies of cultured fibroblasts from patients with type II hyperlipoproteinemia have demonstrated abnormalities of LDL receptors, which, if present throughout the body, could plausibly explain accelerated cholesterol synthesis and limited cholesterol clearance with resultant hypercholesterolemia. Fibroblasts from homozygotes (who have massive hypercholesterolemia and often develop overt arteriosclerotic cardiovascular disease in early childhood) have been found to have no detectable LDL receptors (receptor negative), LDL receptors that bind no more than 10% of the normal number of LDL molecules (receptor defective), or LDL receptors that bind LDL but fail to incorporate LDL into the cell (internalization defect). Fibroblasts from heterozygotes (who have lesser degrees of hypercholesterolemia and develop arteriosclerotic cardiovascular disease at a later age) have been found to have approximately 50% of the normal number of LDL receptors.

It should be emphasized that the type IIa and IIb lipoprotein phenotypes (as well as the type IV phenotype) occur also in familial combined hyperlipoproteinemia, discussed later in this chapter.

TYPE III HYPERLIPOPROTEINEMIA Type III hyperlipoproteinemia is characterized by elevated levels of an intermediate density lipoprotein (IDL). A faint "cream" layer (not chylomicrons) may be seen at the top of refrigerated plasma, and the plasma is usually turbid. Cholesterol and triglyceride levels are both elevated in roughly equal proportions, although the levels are highly variable even in a given patient. An increase in the beta band is seen on lipoprotein electrophoresis (the originally described broad-beta band is seen in approximately two-thirds of patients). Contemporary definitions of type III hyperlipoproteinemia require demonstration of the abnormal lipoprotein ("floating β-VLDL") or of a ratio of VLDL cholesterol to total triglyceride of 0.3 or greater when total triglycerides are between 150 and 1000 mg/100 ml. Both of the latter determinations require ultracentrifugation. Recently, elevated apoprotein E levels (by immunoassay) and absence of an isoprotein of apoprotein E (by isoelectric focusing) have been reported in type III patients. Thus, there is promise of more readily available diagnostic methods for this disorder.

Over one-half of patients with type III hyperlipoproteinemia exhibit planar xanthomas on the palms (xanthoma striata palmaris); tuberous xanthomas are also common. These patients develop premature vascular disease, in general, and have a particularly high incidence of peripheral vascular disease. The vast majority of patients found to have type III hyperlipoproteinemia have been adults. An almost characteristic feature of the disorder is a dramatic response to therapy.

TYPE IV HYPERLIPOPROTEINEMIA Elevated VLDL characterize the type IV pattern. Refrigerated plasma is often turbid, triglyceride levels are elevated, and the pre-beta band is accentuated on lipoprotein electrophoresis.

Type IV hyperlipoproteinemia, a common disorder usually detected in adulthood, is associated with premature vascular disease. Eruptive xanthomas may occur in severely affected patients.

The pathogenesis of type IV hyperlipoproteinemia is unknown. Evidence of accelerated VLDL production and of diminished VLDL clearance in such patients has been reported.

TYPE V HYPERLIPOPROTEINEMIA The combination of elevated VLDL and chylomicrons in plasma from a fasting patient characterizes the type V pattern. A prominent "cream" layer and turbidity of refrigerated plasma, elevated triglyceride levels (with a cholesterol to triglyceride ratio of less than 0.6), and an increase in the pre-beta band and a chylomicron band at the origin on lipoprotein electrophoresis complete the picture.

Although type V patients may have episodes of abdominal pain and hepatomegaly like other patients with hyperchylomicronemia (type I), the type V disorder is usually not expressed until adulthood. Eruptive xanthomas are considerably more common in type V than type IV hyperlipoproteinemia.

COMBINED HYPERLIPOPROTEINEMIA The most recently recognized, and perhaps most common, familial hyperlipoproteinemia is combined hyperlipoproteinemia, which is characterized by the finding of different lipoprotein phenotypes (IIa, IIb, or IV) in different members of the same family. The degree of hyperlipoproteinemia is often modest and not apparent until adult life; xanthomas occur infrequently. The occurrence of premature vascular disease and an association with diabetes are established. The inheritance pattern appears to be autosomal dominant.

PHENOCOPIES The diagnosis of primary hyperlipoproteinemia in the absence of a confirmed familial lipoprotein disorder requires careful exclusion of disorders associated with secondary hyperlipoproteinemia. An attempt has been made to list causes of the various individual lipoprotein patterns in Table 8-3, but it is apparent that these disorders are associated with a variety of patterns. Hypertriglyceridemia and/or hypercholesterolemia occur commonly in diabetes, hypothyroidism, diseases with increased globulin production, acute pancreatitis, and alcoholism. Hypercholesterolemia is a classic, although not invariable, feature of biliary obstruction and the nephrotic syndrome, whereas hypertriglyceridemia has been observed in renal failure, in oral contraceptive use, and in the presence of glucocorticoid excess.

APPROACH TO THE HYPERLIPIDEMIC PATIENT The classification of hyperlipoproteinemia has provided an orderly basis for the evaluation and therapy of hyperlipidemic patients. Along with this advance, lipoprotein electrophoresis is now widely used. It should be apparent from the above discussion that the presence of types I, II, IV, and V can usually be deduced from examination of refrigerated plasma and measurement of serum cholesterol and triglyceride concentrations obtained in the fasting state. Since lipoprotein electrophoresis is not required to diagnose types I, II, IV, and V, and is not diagnostic in type III, its routine use has been seriously questioned.

The uncommon hyperlipidemic patient with chylomicrons observed in refrigerated plasma can be considered to have type I hyperlipoproteinemia if the remainder of the plasma is clear and type V hyperlipoproteinemia if it is turbid. Patients with fasting hyperlipidemia without hyperchylomicronemia will comprise the vast majority of hyperlipidemic patients encountered. Patients with hypercholesterolemia without hypertriglyceridemia have type IIa hyperlipoproteinemia; those with hypertriglyceridemia without hypercholesterolemia have type IV hyperlipoproteinemia. The remainder, with "mixed hyperlipidemia" (elevation of both cholesterol and triglycerides), can usually be tentatively classified as follows: a cholesterol to triglyceride ratio greater than 1.5 suggests type IIb hyperlipoproteinemia, predominant hypertriglyceridemia suggests type IV hyperlipoproteinemia, and hypercholesterolemia and hypertriglyceridemia of roughly equal proportions raises the possibility of type III hyperlipoproteinemia. Under optimal circumstances, serum ultracentrifugation should be employed for all patients with mixed hyperlipidemia. A practical compromise, however, is to use the rules outlined and obtain ultracentrifugation studies when these and/or clinical considerations—planar (especially on the palms) or tuberous xanthomas and/or occlusive peripheral vascular disease—make type III hyperlipoproteinemia a reasonable possibility.

SUGGESTED READING

1. Frederickson DS, Goldstein JL, Brown MS: The familial hyperlipoproteinemias. *In* The Metabolic Basis of Inherited Disease, Fourth Edition. Stanbury JB, Wyngaarden JB, Fredrickson DS (eds). McGraw-Hill, New York, 1978, p 604.
2. Fisher WR, Truitt DH: The common hyperlipoproteinemias. *Ann Intern Med* 85:497, 1976.
3. Gordon T, Castelli WP, Hjortland MC, Kannel WB, Dawber TR: High density lipoprotein as a protective factor against coronary heart disease. *Amer J Med* 62:707, 1977.
4. Goldstein JL, Brown MS: The low-density lipoprotein pathway and its relation to atherosclerosis. *Ann Rev Biochem* 46:897, 1977.
5. Small DM: Cellular mechanisms for lipid deposition in atherosclerosis. *N Engl J Med* 297:873 and 924, 1977.
6. Mann GV: Diet-Heart: End of an era. *N Engl J Med* 297:644, 1977.
7. Glueck CJ, Mattson F, Bierman EL: Diet and coronary heart disease: Another view. *N Engl J Med* 298:1471, 1978.
8. Barndt R Jr, Blankenhorn DH, Crawford DW, Brooks SH: Regression and progression of early femoral atherosclerosis in treated hyperlipoproteinemic patients. *Ann Intern Med* 86:139, 1977.
9. Kushwaha RS, Hazzard WR, Wahl PW, Hoover JJ: Type III hyperlipoproteinemia: Diagnosis in whole plasma by apolipoprotein-E immunoassay. *Ann Intern Med* 86:509, 1977.
10. Greenberg BH, Blackwelder WC, Levy RI: Primary type V hyperlipoproteinemia. A descriptive study in 32 families. *Ann Intern Med* 87:526, 1977.

9

HYPERGLYCEMIA AND HYPOGLYCEMIA

Certain tissues, notably those of the central nervous system, are dependent on a continuous supply of glucose. The plasma glucose concentration is normally maintained within rather narrow limits whether the individual is feeding or fasting. This is accomplished by hormonal, and perhaps neural, modulation of glucose influx into the circulation and glucose efflux from the circulation. During feeding, glucose utilization and glucose storage (glycogen synthesis) accelerate, while endogenous glucose formation (glycogenolysis, gluconeogenesis) diminishes. During fasting, glucose utilization by such tissues as the brain continues but that by other tissues declines, and endogenous glucose formation (glycogenolysis, gluconeogenesis) accelerates.* These changes are summarized schematically in Fig. 9-1.

Insulin is the primary modulator of glucose homeostasis. During feeding, insulin stimulates glucose utilization by insulin-sensitive tissues (such as muscle and fat) and glycogen synthesis; it suppresses gluconeogenesis. During fasting, insulin levels drop, stimulating increased glucose production (gluconeogenesis, decreased

* The normal adult has an obligatory glucose requirement of 150 to 180 gm daily, of which approximately 80% is utilized by the central nervous system. Since this requirement is approximately twice the amount of glucose that can be generated from hepatic glycogen stores, the fasting individual is critically dependent on new glucose formation via gluconeogenesis.

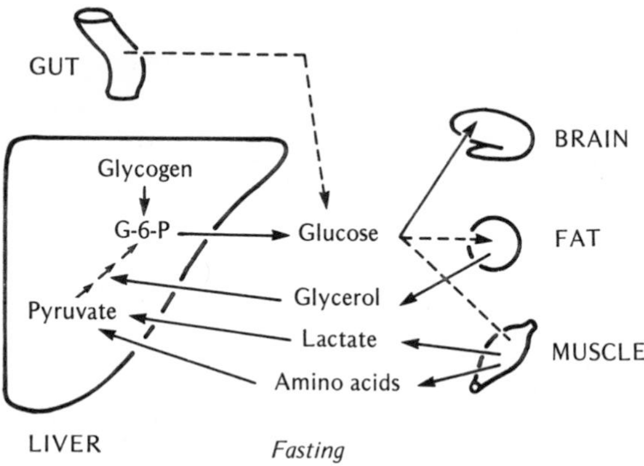

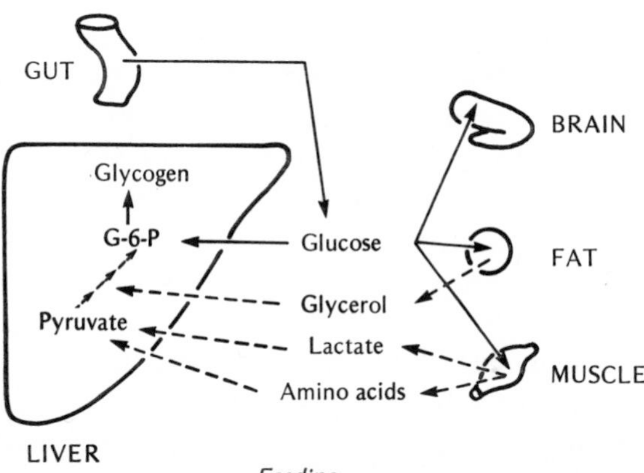

FIG. 9-1. Overview of the metabolic adaptation to fasting and feeding as it relates to glucose homeostasis.

glycogen synthesis) and decreased glucose utilization by insulin-sensitive tissues. In recent years, an important role for glucagon, particularly with respect to the regulation of hepatic glucose production, has been suggested. Thus, during feeding, high insulin to glucagon ratios favor glycogen synthesis and diminished gluconeogenesis; during fasting, low insulin to glucagon ratios favor glycogenolysis and gluconeogenesis. Several other hormones, such as epinephrine, cortisol, and growth hormone (and the neurotransmitter norepinephrine), can, either directly or indirectly, elevate the plasma glucose concentration. How these factors, relative to insulin and glucagon, contribute to the maintenance of normal glucose homeostasis remains to be defined, but their excess or deficit can lead to overt distortion of glucose homeostasis.

Factors that alter the secretion of insulin and glucagon are summarized in Table 9-1. Despite the multiple factors involved in the regulation of insulin (and glucagon) secretion, it is conceptually sound to view the plasma glucose concentration as the primary regulated variable and, thus, the prime determinant of the secretion of these hormones. An increase in the plasma glucose level triggers insulin release; insulin secretion falls to low levels when the plasma glucose concentration falls to approximately 60 mg/100 ml or less. Hypoglycemia triggers glucagon release; hyperglycemia may suppress glucagon secretion. Autonomic (adrenergic and cholinergic) modulation of insulin secretion is well established, and adrenergic influences on glucagon secretion have been demonstrated. The augmented insulin response to oral, as opposed to intravenous, glucose has been attributed to the release of gastrointestinal hormones(which stimulate insulin secretion) after oral glucose.

Disorders of glucose homeostasis resulting in hyperglycemia are common, particularly genetic diabetes mellitus. Although the incidence of hypoglycemia is unknown, in part because there is no widely accepted definition of it, spontaneous symptomatic hypoglycemia is uncommon.

ANALYTICAL METHODS

With automated methodology, plasma glucose concentrations can be measured rapidly with more than adequate analytical precision. A ferricyanide method has been widely used with automated equipment. With this method, a variety of non-glucose reducing substances (including creatinine and bilirubin) can cause artifactual elevation of the "glucose" determination. The more specific

Table 9-1

Factors affecting insulin and glucagon secretion.
All are stimulatory except as noted

A. Insulin Secretion
- 1. Metabolic fuels
  - a. Glucose (an increase in plasma glucose stimulates insulin secretion; a decrease in plasma glucose suppresses insulin secretion)
  - b. Amino acids (e.g., arginine, leucine)
- 2. Autonomic influences
  - a. Adrenergic (alpha-adrenergic stimulation decreases insulin secretion; beta-adrenergic stimulation increases insulin secretion)
  - b. Cholinergic
- 3. Gut hormones
  - a. Cholescystokinin-pancreozymin
  - b. Secretin
  - c. Gastrin
  - d. Glucagon
- 4. Other hormones
  - a. Direct and indirect–Glucagon
  - b. Probably indirect–Growth hormone, glucocorticoids, estrogens, parathyroid hormone

B. Glucagon Secretion
- 1. Metabolic fuels
  - a. Glucose (hypoglycemia stimulates glucagon secretion; hyperglycemia may suppress glucagon secretion)
  - b. Amino acids (e.g., arginine, alanine)
- 2. Autonomic influences
  - Adrenergic
- 3. Gut hormones
  - a. Pancreozymin
  - b. ? Secretin

glucose oxidase method has more recently been adapted to automated equipment and is preferable.

Whole blood glucose determinations have been largely replaced by plasma (or serum) glucose measurements. Due to the relatively low glucose content of the cellular components of whole blood, plasma (or serum) glucose concentrations are roughly 15% higher than whole blood glucose concentrations. Delayed separation of plasma from the formed elements of the blood can result in an appreciable reduction in the plasma glucose concentration due to continued glucose utilization by the blood cells. This can be avoided by prompt separation of the plasma and greatly limited by refrigeration of the sample before separation and also by addition of an inhibitor of glycolysis, such as sodium fluoride. Since fluoride in high concentration can interfere with glucose oxidase methods, a maximum sodium fluoride concentration of 2 mg/ml is recommended. At this concentration, sodium fluoride is not an effective anticoagulant, and an additional agent, such as EDTA, is often added.

Although quantitative measurements of urine glucose are infrequently performed, qualitative or semiquantitative measurements of urine glucose are widely used. Again, the more specific glucose oxidase methods, which are available in "dipstick" form (e.g., Diastix, Ames), are preferable.

Quantitative methods for the measurement of "ketone bodies" (acetoacetate, β-hydroxybutyrate) are not generally available for clinical use. A qualitative nitroprusside method, however, is readily available in the form of tablets (e.g., Acetest, Ames), dipsticks (e.g., Ketostix, Ames), or powder (e.g., Denco Acetone Test Powder, Denver Chemical Manufacturing). These can be used with urine or serum, often semiquantitatively, by testing serial dilutions of serum. It should be emphasized that the nitroprusside reagent primarily detects acetoacetate. Thus, appreciable "ketosis" in the form of β-hydroxybutyrate can be present with a negative nitroprusside reaction.

The radioimmunoassay concept arose from the measurement of insulin in plasma, and insulin radioimmunoassays are widely available. Insulin antisera cross-react with the precursor hormone proinsulin, which circulates in plasma and has very little biologic activity relative to insulin. During fasting, plasma insulin may fall to levels that are at the lower limit of assay sensitivity; thus, low insulin levels should be interpreted with caution and, preferably, with a knowledge of the precision of the particular assay used. Since insulin-treated patients develop antibodies to insulin, radioimmunoassays of plasma insulin, for all practical purposes, cannot be performed in such patients. Radioimmunoassay of C-peptide (the peptide chain removed from proinsulin during its conversion to insulin) has been used as an index of insulin secretion in insulin-treated patients, but C-peptide antiserum is not widely available, except in research laboratories.

Other hormones relevant to the regulation of glucose homeostasis can also be measured by radioimmunoassay. Plasma glucagon levels have been extensively studied in several research laboratories, but glucagon radioimmunoassays are not yet generally available. Several difficulties in the interpretation of glucagon immunoassay results have arisen. Some of the initial antiserums were found to react not only with glucagon of pancreatic origin but also with a material of gastrointestinal origin ("gut glucagon" or glucagon-like immunoreactivity, GLI). More recently, antiserums believed to be specific for pancreatic glucagon (i.e., they showed no cross-reactivity with gut glucagon) have detected readily measurable plasma glucagon levels in totally pancreatectomized animals. It has now been shown that glucagon indistinguishable from pancreatic glucagon arises from extrapancreatic sites, including the gastrointestinal tract. Nonetheless, plasma glucagon assays have been of value in certain rare clinical disorders, notably the detection of glucagon-secreting pancreatic islet cell tumors. Measurements of plasma catecholamines, growth hormone, and cortisol, all of which affect glucose homeostasis, have been discussed earlier.

HYPERGLYCEMIA

Diabetes mellitus is a common disease affecting between 1 and 5% of the population. Diabetes is a complex genetic and environmental disorder involving alterations of carbohydrate, protein, and fat metabolism and the development of microvascular disease (characterized by thickening of the capillary basement membranes), neuropathy, and macrovascular disease, indistinguishable from atherosclerotic disease in nondiabetics. Nonetheless, as a practical matter, the diagnosis of diabetes mellitus is based upon the demonstration of hyperglycemia either in the fasting state or in response to a glucose challenge.

Although the pathogenesis of genetic diabetes is a matter of some debate, defects in insulin secretion have been demonstrated in a large number of diabetic patients by several groups of investigators. These range from a slight impairment of early insulin release in patients with a genetic predisposition to diabetes but normal glucose tolerance tests to absolute insulin deficiency in patients with severe, persistent hyperglycemia. Evidence indicating that resistance to the effects of insulin (i.e., decreased glucose utilization, increased glucose production, or both inappropriate to the ambient insulin concentration) occurs in a variety of disorders associated with glucose intolerance, including diabetes mellitus, has been presented, and a fascinating array of mechanisms have been proposed. Whether such insulin resistance can produce glucose intolerance in the absence of a defect in insulin secretion is currently not known, although evidence for either point of view can be cited. In the author's judgment, insulin resistance probably does produce glucose intolerance, although it uncommonly produces fasting hyperglycemia and symptomatic diabetes in the absence of an associated defect in insulin secretion. As a practical matter, measurement of serum insulin concentrations is of little value in the clinical evaluation of patients with suspected or proven diabetes.

Various clinical classifications of diabetic patients have been proposed. That suggested by Renold, Muller, Mintz, and Cahill (and, of previous classifications, most similar to that of the British Diabetes Association) is outlined in Table 9-2. It should be emphasized that progression through these classes, although it may well occur, is not predictable in a given patient. Many patients retain the lesser glucose abnormalities for years or even decades, and regression from greater to lesser degrees of glucose intolerance is well documented, particularly after weight reduction.

Table 9-2
Clinical classification of patients with diabetes mellitus

A. Potential Diabetes–Birth to the onset of glucose intolerance. Diagnosable only in retrospect

B. Latent Diabetes–Transient glucose intolerance during stress (e.g., during pregnancy)

C. Chemical Diabetes–Glucose intolerance with normal or only slightly elevated fasting plasma glucose concentrations

D. Overt Diabetes–Persistent fasting hyperglycemia. May be further subclassified:
   1. Insulin independent
   2. Insulin dependent

A discussion of recent developments in the field of diabetes, such as the interplay between genetic and environmental factors (HLA association, the possible role of viral infection and islet cell antibodies) and the possible roles of altered insulin receptors and of glucagon in the pathogenesis of the disease are beyond the scope of this book, although references to these topics are listed at the end of this chapter. Several points should, however, be made. First, genetic heterogeneity has now been recognized in diabetes. For example, glucose intolerance in young patients ("maturity onset diabetes of the young") appears to be inherited as a dominant disorder, whereas the inheritance of overt, insulin dependent, ketosis prone diabetes ("juvenile diabetes") more closely approximates that of a recessive trait. Second, nonenzymatic glycosylation of proteins occurs in hyperglycemic patients. For example, overtly diabetic patients have increased proportions of glycosylated hemoglobins (e.g., hemoglobin A_{1c}). Since these hemoglobins, once glycosylated, persist in the circulation for the life-span of the red blood cell, measurement of glycosylated hemoglobin levels may well provide an index of the integrated degree of hyperglycemia over several weeks and, thus, provide a useful measure of the adequacy of glucose control in a given patient. When compared to oral glucose tolerance testing, however, measurement of the glycosylated hemoglobin level does not provide diagnostic sensitivity, although it could be argued that it does provide biologically relevant information. Third, although still a matter of debate, it appears to the author that the weight of evidence favors the conclusion that capillary basement membrane thickening is an acquired feature of diabetes rather than a primary pathogenic feature of the disease.

Symptoms directly attributable to the metabolic abnormality of diabetes mellitus include polyuria (osmotic diuresis due to glycosuria), with polydipsia and weight loss (inadequate assimilation of metabolic fuels) despite polyphagia. Others include blurred vision, recurrent infections, and nonspecific malaise. Diabetic microangiopathy is most prominently reflected in the development of retinopathy, nephropathy, and disease of the distal lower extremities. Diabetic retinopathy can be subdivided into background retinopathy (e.g., microaneurysms, small hemorrhages, and exudates), which generally does not, in itself, threaten vision, and proliferative retinopathy (neovascularization), which is a serious threat to vision and a relatively common cause of blindness. Cataracts can also impair vision in diabetics. Diabetic glomerulosclerosis, usually associated with recognizable retinopathy, may cause massive proteinuria and renal failure. Pyelonephritis and nephrosclerosis are common concomitants of diabetic glomerulosclerosis. Peripheral microangiopathy can lead to patchy gangrene of distal portions of the lower extremities. Atherosclerotic macrovascular disease of the coronary arteries is the most common cause of death in diabetics. Atherosclerotic cerebrovascular disease and peripheral vascular disease also occur commonly. Although a symmetrical, distal, predominantly sensory neuropathy is the most common expression of diabetic somatic neuropathy, a large variety of patterns are seen. Visceral (autonomic) neuropathy can cause manifestations such as postural hypotension, impotence, diarrhea, and gastric dilation, among others.

Normal subjects generally have *fasting plasma glucose* concentrations of 70 to 110 mg/100 ml. When the fasting value is reproducibly and unequivocally elevated (e.g., over 130 mg/100 ml on at least two occasions), the patient has the carbohydrate abnormality of overt diabetes. A glucose tolerance test is superfluous in such a patient. When the fasting plasma glucose concentration is normal (and diabetes is suspected for other reasons) or borderline high, a glucose tolerance test is in order.

The *oral glucose tolerance test* is performed after an overnight fast, preferably in ambulatory patients, in the absence of major stress and after a period of relatively high carbohydrate intake. Dietary carbohydrate restriction can result in impaired glucose tolerance and an erroneous (by current criteria) diagnosis of diabetes. A minimum carbohydrate intake of 300 gm daily for at least 3 days before the test is often recommended, although the American Diabetes Association recommendation is for a minimum of 150 gm of carbohydrate daily for 3 days before the test. The approximate carbohydrate content of some common foods that can be used to augment dietary carbohydrate intake before a glucose tolerance test is listed in Table 9-3. Since some diurnal variation in glucose tolerance has been described, the test should be performed in the morning. The patient should avoid undue physical activity, smoking, and coffee drinking during the test.

Several sets of criteria for interpretation of the oral glucose tolerance test have been proposed; two are shown in Table 9-4. The differences between these is perhaps partially explained by the use of a larger glucose dose (1.75 gm/kg of body weight) in the studies of Andres. A glucose load of 40 gm/m^2 of body surface area has been recommended, although many physicians use fixed doses of 75 or 100 gm of glucose for oral glucose testing. The minimum sampling times for plasma glucose measurements are at zero time (before glucose) and at 60 and 120 minutes after glucose ingestion. If reactive hypoglycemia is suspected (see below), the test should be extended to 300 minutes, and samples should be drawn at 30-minute intervals.

The following points should be emphasized in interpreting an oral glucose tolerance test:

1. As is apparent from the age adjustments in Table 9-4, it is now

Table 9-3

Approximate carbohydrate content of common foods, which can be used to ensure adequate carbohydrate intake before a glucose tolerance test (prepared by the dietary staff of the Washington University School of Medicine Clinical Research Center)

LIST I (any one contains approximately 15 gm of carbohydrate)

1 slice bread or 1 soft dinner roll	1¼ cup milk
1 baking powder biscuit	½ cup ice cream
1 plain or sugar doughnut	1 brownie (2 × 2 × ¾ inch)
1 muffin	2 cookies
1 oz or 15 medium potato chips	1-oz chocolate bar
1 medium apple	1 tbsp jelly or honey
1 medium orange	2 rounded tsp sugar

LIST II (any one item contains approximately 25 gm of carbohydrate)

1 cup chocolate milk	¾ cup lima beans
1 cup cooked or dry cereal	½ cup regular canned fruit
1 medium potato or 1 cup mashed	½ cup sherbet
¾ cup corn	½ cup vanilla pudding

LIST III (any one item contains approximately 35 gm of carbohydrate)

1 cup cooked macaroni, noodles, or rice	1 piece cake with icing
1 large banana	⅛ of 9-inch pie
12-oz soft drink	½ cup chocolate or butterscotch pudding
1 sweet roll or jelly doughnut	

well established that glucose tolerance deteriorates with advancing age. The post-glucose plasma glucose concentration increases approximately 8 to 13 mg/100 ml per decade of adult life.* From the extensive data of Andres, one would predict that approximately 70% of 80-year-olds would have a plasma glucose concen-

* In contrast, the fasting plasma glucose level increases only about 2 mg/100 ml per decade of adult life.

Table 9-4
Upper limits of "normal" for oral glucose tolerance testing

AGE (YEARS)	FAJANS 0	60	120	SUM	ANDRES 0	60	120	SUM
0–30	110	185	140	435	110	185	165	460
30–40	110	185	140	435	112	191	175	478
40-50	110	185	140	435	114	197	185	496
50–60	110	195	150	455	116	203	195	514
60–70	110	205	160	475	118	209	205	532
70–80	110	215	170	495	120	215	215	550

tration greater than 140 mg/100 ml 2 hours after an oral glucose load of 1.75 gm/kg body weight. Thus, the diagnosis of diabetes mellitus based upon glucose intolerance alone is particularly treacherous in older members of the population.

2. With one recognized exception (the Pima Indians), the distribution of glucose tolerance patterns in the population is not bimodal but rather represents a spectrum from "normal" to "abnormal." Thus, the limits of normality are, of necessity, arbitrary.

3. As mentioned earlier, an abnormal glucose tolerance test does not indicate that clinically overt, symptomatic diabetes mellitus is inevitable. Progression, although it does occur, is not predictable, and regression to normal glucose tolerance has been described.

4. Glucose intolerance occurs in a variety of disorders other than genetic diabetes, as summarized in Table 9-5. In patients with any of these disorders, it is often impossible to determine whether or not genetic diabetes mellitus, a common disorder, is also present.

In view of the reservations cited, conservatism in the diagnosis of diabetes mellitus based on a mildly abnormal glucose tolerance test alone is appropriate. What service is done to the patient with a normal fasting plasma glucose concentration and no evidence of typical vascular lesions by labeling him "diabetic," because of an abnormal glucose tolerance test? Specific, curative therapy is not available, and general therapeutic recommendations, such as

Table 9-5
Disorders associated with glucose intolerance

A. Genetic Diabetes Mellitus

B. Pancreatic Damage
   1. Pancreatectomy
   2. Chronic pancreatitis
   3. Pancreatic carcinoma
   4. Iron overload
   5. Cystic fibrosis

C. Classic Endocrine Hyperfunction
   1. Glucocorticoid and/or mineralocorticoid excess (Cushing's syndrome, aldosteronism)
   2. Catecholamine excess (pheochromocytoma)
   3. Growth hormone excess (acromegaly)
   4. Glucagon excess (pancreatic islet cell tumors)
   5. Parathyroid hormone excess (hyperparathyroidism)
   6. Thyroid hormone excess (hyperthyroidism)

D. Other[a]
   1. Renal insufficiency
   2. Hepatic disease
   3. Low carbohydrate intake
   4. Pregnancy
   5. Drugs–glucocorticoids, estrogens, thiazides, diphenylhydantoin, salicylates, nicotinic acid
   6. Stress
   7. Miscellaneous–chronic decreased cardiac output, Huntington's chorea, myotonic dystrophy, etc.

[a] It is likely that hormonal mechanisms participate in the pathogenesis of glucose intolerance in several of these disorders.

weight reduction for the obese patient, can be made in good conscience without a diagnosis of diabetes. The absence of a dogmatic diagnosis of diabetes should not be a barrier to education of the patient concerning the manifestations of diabetes or to careful medical follow-up so that progression, if it occurs, can be detected and, if necessary, treated.

The *intravenous glucose tolerance test* is useful when difficulties with glucose ingestion, transport within the upper gastrointestinal tract, or absorption are anticipated, as in a patient who has had gastric surgery. In general, the precautions described for the oral test also apply to the intravenous test. Various glucose doses have been used. A fixed dose of 25 gm is convenient; a dose of 0.5 gm/kg body weight is conceptually more attractive although not of proven superiority. Glucose is infused over 4 minutes or less, and plasma samples for glucose determinations are obtained 10, 20, 30, 40, 50, and 60 minutes after the mid-injection time. The plasma glucose levels are then plotted on a semilogarithmic plot against time. A straight line best fitting the points is drawn, and the time (in minutes) required for the plasma glucose to fall by 50% ($t\frac{1}{2}$) is read off. A k value (glucose disappearance rate in percent per minute) is then calculated as follows:

$$k = \frac{0.693}{t\frac{1}{2}} \times 100$$

Patients with diabetes have lower k values than normal subjects have. The normal intravenous glucose tolerance test has been less well defined than the normal oral glucose tolerance test. Some regard values greater than 1.10 as normal, values lower than 0.90 as abnormal (diabetic), and values from 0.90 to 1.10 as borderline. Others consider the borderline range to be higher (e.g., 1.20 to 1.29). Intravenous glucose tolerance, like oral glucose tolerance, deteriorates with age.

Glycosuria, although indicative of diabetes in most cases, is not itself sufficient evidence for a diagnosis of diabetes. The renal "threshold" for escape of glucose into the urine varies widely, and postprandial glycosuria occasionally is detected in patients who cannot be shown to have diabetes by glucose tolerance testing. The uncommon finding of fasting glycosuria associated with normal fasting plasma glucose concentrations ("renal glycosuria") does not indicate that diabetes will develop in the future.

Diabetic ketoacidosis can be viewed as a state of absolute insulin deficiency. Glucose production is accelerated, and glucose utilization is decreased, resulting in major hyperglycemia and glycosuria; the resulting osmotic diuresis leads to electrolyte depletion and volume contraction. If the latter appreciably reduces renal function, the capacity to excrete glucose is limited, and massive hyperglycemia may result. Accelerated lipolysis and ketone body formation, resulting in ketoacidosis, complete the picture of absolute insulin deficiency. If the available insulin is sufficient to prevent accelerated lipolysis and ketogenesis but insufficient to inhibit glucose production and stimulate glucose utilization, hyperglycemia without ketosis results; the development of impaired renal function under these conditions can lead to massive hyperglycemia—the *non-ketotic hyperosmolar syndrome.*

Patients with diabetic ketoacidosis exhibit a variety of nonspecific symptoms. Nausea is common. Clinically apparent hyperpnea (Kussmaul's respiration) generally implies an arterial pH less than 7.20. Progressive impairment of central nervous system function occurs with severe ketoacidosis. The clinical manifestations of an underlying, precipitating illness may be apparent. Patients with the non-ketotic hyperosmolar syndrome are often severely volume contracted and generally have prominent central nervous system impairment.

Diabetic ketosis is diagnosed when glycosuria, ketonuria, and ketonemia are demonstrated. Additional studies define the severity of the disorder (arterial pH or venous bicarbonate, semiquantification of ketonemia by study of serial dilutions of serum) and establish base-line chemistries (serum glucose, electrolytes, urea nitrogen, etc.). It should be recalled that the nitroprusside reagent used to measure serum ketone bodies detects acetoacetate (not β-hydroxybutyrate). Thus, if the redox state favors the formation of reduced compounds, serum "ketones" may not be strikingly elevated despite severe ketoacidosis. In patients with severe ketoacidosis, lactic acidosis may also contribute to the depressed arterial pH. In the absence of ketonemia, the diabetic with impaired central nervous system function may be hypoglycemic or severely hyperglycemic (non-ketotic hyperosmolar syndrome).

HYPOGLYCEMIA

The central nervous system is critically dependent on glucose as an energy substrate and cannot extract glucose from the plasma against a concentration gradient. Therefore, very low plasma glucose concentrations can cause severe dysfunction of the central nervous system and death.

The clinical manifestations of hypoglycemia are often divided into two categories, those attributable to the sympathetic discharge triggered by acute hypoglycemia and those attributable to central nervous system dysfunction due to glucose deprivation per se. Tachycardia, palpitations, and diaphoresis are typical sympathetic manifestations. Anxiety, hunger, and weakness are often included in this category. In general, these symptoms are associated with a rapid fall in the plasma glucose concentration to hypoglycemic levels. The sympathetic manifestations are often absent when hypoglycemia develops insidiously. Furthermore, sympathetic symptoms during acute hypoglycemia (e.g., an insulin reaction) become progressively less prominent in some patients with long-standing diabetes.

Clinically, central nervous system glucose deprivation spans a broad spectrum from subtle impairment of mentation to death. Acute and transient hypoglycemia may be associated with headache, visual symptoms, lethargy, confusion, an inappropriate affect, etc. Severe, prolonged hypoglycemia may be associated with coma and death. Between these extremes, a variety of symptoms including lack of coordination, impairment of sensory and motor function, irrational behavior, and dementia may occur. Seizures, which are unusual in spontaneously hypoglycemic adults, are often a clue to the presence of hypoglycemia in children. Hypothermia due to hypoglycemia has been well documented. Post-hypoglycemic fever has been more recently described.

Recovery from hypoglycemic central nervous system dysfunction is typically prompt with restoration of the plasma glucose concentration to normal. Recovery may be delayed, however, after severe, prolonged hypoglycemia. In some instances, reversible coma persists for days, despite normalization of the plasma glucose level. Permanent brain damage had been attributed to recurrent bouts of hypoglycemia.

Simply stated, the plasma glucose concentration is the resultant of glucose influx into the circulation and glucose efflux out of the circulation. Normally, cessation of glucose influx from the gastrointestinal tract, acceleration of glucose efflux into the tissues, or both are compensated for by an increase in the flow of endogenous glucose into the circulation from the liver (glycogenolysis, gluconeogenesis). This compensatory response requires:

1. An intact hormonal, and possibly neural, regulatory response. The plasma glucagon, cortisol, growth hormone, epinephrine, and norepinephrine responses to (insulin-induced) hypoglycemia are illustrated in Fig. 9-2. Of these, it is the author's opinion, based upon recent studies, that glucagon is particularly critical to recovery from hypoglycemia, that epinephrine can compensate for glucagon lack, and that the others are less important in recovery from acute hypoglycemia. They may well, however, play a more important role in the prevention of fasting hypoglycemia.
2. Structural and enzymatic integrity of the hepatic glycogenolytic and gluconeogenic systems.
3. Mobilization and transport of gluconeogenic substrates, such as amino acids, lactate, and glycerol to the liver.

Failure of these mechanisms to fully compensate for a falling plasma glucose concentration results in hypoglycemia.

It is clinically convenient to divide patients with hypoglycemia into two broad categories:

1. Reactive hypoglycemia–hypoglycemia within approximately 5 hours of food ingestion.
2. Fasting hypoglycemia–hypoglycemia after the patient passes from the fed to the fasted state.

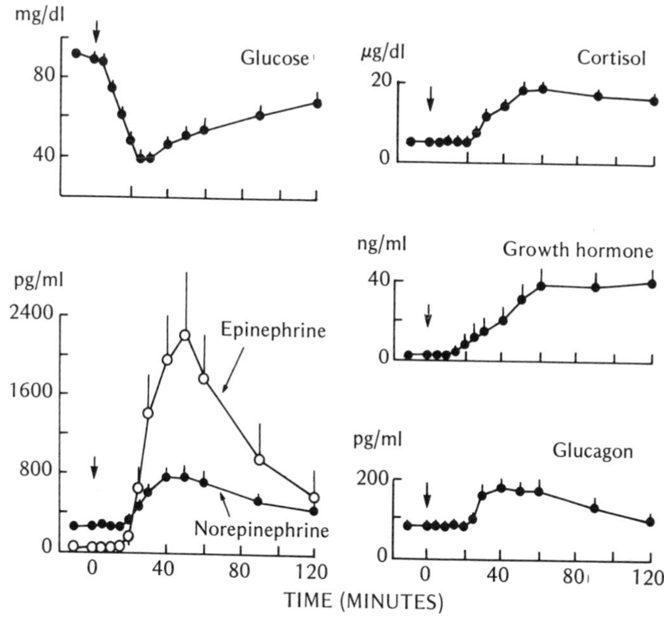

FIG. 9-2. Mean (± S.E.) plasma glucose, epinephrine, norepinephrine, cortisol, growth hormone, and glucagon responses to insulin-induced hypoglycemia (0.15 units of regular insulin/kg body weight, arrows) in six normal male subjects. (Adapted from data presented in Garber AJ, Cryer PE, Santiago JV et al: *J Clin Invest* 58:7, 1976.)

The first question to be answered about patients with proven or suspected hypoglycemia is whether or not they have fasting hypoglycemia, since fasting hypoglycemia is generally indicative of a serious underlying disorder and is often life-threatening in itself, and since patients with fasting hypoglycemia may also have reactive hypoglycemia. Once the presence of fasting hypoglycemia is established, the differential diagnosis becomes that of fasting hypoglycemia irrespective of the presence or absence of reactive hypoglycemia. If fasting hypoglycemia can be confidently excluded, and reactive hypoglycemia is present, the differential diagnosis can be greatly narrowed.

Fasting hypoglycemia is an uncommon disorder. It is discussed in some detail in this chapter because of its serious implications, not because of its frequency. Various causes of fasting hypoglycemia are listed in Table 9-6. This disorder often results from decreased glucose production plus increased glucose utilization. Since obligate glucose utilization continues during fasting, decreased glucose production alone can produce fasting hypoglycemia. But, it has not been established that increased glucose utilization alone, in the absence of a defect in glucose production, causes hypoglycemia. In this sense, then, the three categories listed in Table 9-6 are somewhat artificial.

Drugs, particularly alcohol and the hypoglycemic drugs prescribed for patients with diabetes, are a relatively common cause of fasting hypoglycemia. A variety of other drugs (listed in Table 9-6) have been associated with hypoglycemia, but in most cases, other factors contribute to the development of hypoglycemia. Alcohol limits gluconeogenesis. Alcoholic hypoglycemia usually occurs only when limited food intake is coupled with heavy alcohol ingestion. Clearly, this combination may be seen in binge drinkers as well as daily heavy drinkers. Since plasma glucose concentration lowering is the desired pharmacologic effect of insulin and the oral hypoglycemic drugs, hypoglycemia can result from accidental or intentional overdosage of these drugs. In addition, hypoglycemia can occur in patients taking a constant dose of a hypoglycemic drug, if other states that favor decreased glucose production, such as renal failure, develop. Lastly, the surreptitious use of hypoglycemic drugs should be considered in a patient with unexplained hypoglycemia, especially if the patient has a knowledge of these drugs and access to them.

Hormonal deficits constitute a well-defined category of causes of hypoglycemia. Of the various deficiency states, glucocorticoid deficiency is most consistently associated with fasting hypoglycemia. Nonetheless, the majority of glucocorticoid-deficient adults are not hypoglycemic. In general, hormonal deficiency states more often cause hypoglycemia in children than in adults. Hypoglycemia has been recognized in patients with isolated growth hormone deficiency, but it is more likely if both ACTH and growth hormone secretion are deficient. Hypoglycemia has been attributed to hypothyroidism. An impaired epinephrine response has been demonstrated in some hypoglycemic patients, but a cause and effect relationship has not been established. Although catecholamine lack may play a role in the pathogenesis of hypoglycemia, it is noteworthy that hypoglycemia does not regularly occur in cortisol-substituted adrenalectomized patients or in patients with extensive degenerative disease of the autonomic nervous system. Hypoglycemia has also been attributed to glucagon deficiency.

Hypoglycemia due to generalized liver disease is seen only with the destruction of more than 80% of the liver. Liver disease is, therefore, clinically overt in such patients. Although glucose intolerance is well known in uremic patients, the development of fasting hypoglycemia in patients with renal failure has been recognized only recently. Kinetic studies in a single patient with chronic renal failure have been interpreted as indicating that the patient's fasting hypoglycemia was due to inadequate mobilization of gluconeogenic substrate ("substrate-limited gluconeogenesis"), a mechanism believed to underlie the development of hypoglycemia in the ketotic hypoglycemia syndrome of childhood. The latter, perhaps the most common cause of hypoglycemia in children, is believed to be a self-limited disorder, which does not

Table 9-6
Causes of fasting hypoglycemia

A. Decreased Glucose Production Predominant
   1. Drugs[a]
      a. Alcohol
      b. Phenformin
      c. Salicylates
      d. (Insulin)
      e. (Sulfonylureas)
   2. Hormonal deficits
      a. Glucocorticoids
      b. Growth hormone
      c. Thyroid hormones

Table 9-6 Continued

- d. ? Catecholamines
- e. ? Glucagon

3. Extensive hepatic destruction
4. Chronic renal failure
5. Ketotic hypoglycemia of childhood
6. Congenital enzyme defects[b]
7. Neonatal hypoglycemia
   - a. Premature infants
   - b. Small-for-gestational-age infants

B. Increased Glucose Utilization Predominant

1. Extrapancreatic tumors
2. Pregnancy
3. Severe exercise
4. Renal glycosuria

C. Decreased Glucose Production and Increased Glucose Utilization

1. Hyperinsulinism
   - a. Pancreatic β-cell disorders–tumor, hyperplasia, nesidioblastosis, functional (including "leucine sensitivity")
   - b. Exogenous insulin or sulfonylureas
   - c. Neonatal hypoglycemia in infants or diabetic mothers, erythroblastosis fetalis
2. Extrapancreatic tumors that secrete compounds with biologic activity similar to insulin (e.g., NSILA)

---

[a] Hypoglycemia has been attributed to various additional drugs including propranolol, oxytetracycline, monoamine oxidase inhibitors, EDTA, para-aminobenzoate, haloperidol, chlorpromazine, and propoxyphene.

[b] The prototypes of the congenital enzyme defects that cause hypoglycemia are deficiencies of the enzyme required for hepatic glucose release (glucose-6-phosphatase deficiency, glycogen storage disease type I) or of enzymes required for gluconeogenesis (e.g., fructose-1,6-diphosphatase deficiency). Typically, these deficiencies produce profound hypoglycemia with hepatomegaly and a catastrophic clinical illness seen in infancy. Although pyruvate carboxylase deficiency would be expected to cause defective gluconeogenesis, major hypoglycemia has not been recognized in patients believed to be deficient in this enzyme. Enzyme defects that impair glycogen synthesis (glycogen synthetase deficiency) or glycogenolysis (amylo-1,6-glucosidase deficiency, glycogen storage disease type III and "phosphorylase" deficiency, glycogen storage disease type VI) have less striking effects on the plasma glucose concentration, although fasting hypoglycemia may occur. In contrast to these enzyme deficiencies that cause fasting hypoglycemia, deficiencies of galactose-1-phosphate uridyl transferase (galactosemia) and of fructose-1-phosphate aldolase (hereditary fructose intolerance) cause postprandial (reactive) hypoglycemia.

persist into adult life. In contrast, congenital enzyme defects in hepatic glucose production generally produce a catastrophic clinical illness that includes hypoglycemia early in life.

Hypoglycemia at times occurs in patients with extrapancreatic tumors. Such tumors are often quite large, even massive, and there is evidence that they utilize large quantities of glucose. Whether or not any of these tumors produce hypoglycemia due only to increased glucose utilization remains to be established. Production of a humoral substance with hypoglycemic biologic activity from such tumors has been widely suspected, but serum immunoreactive insulin levels have been uniformly (appropriately) low. The recent demonstration of radioreceptor assayable, nonsuppressible insulin-like activity (NSILA-s)* in the serum of several patients with hypoglycemia and extrapancreatic tumors lends further support to this concept. Other conditions associated with increased glucose utilization and/or excretion, such as exercise, pregnancy, and renal glycosuria, rarely if ever cause hypoglycemia unless defects in glucose formation also occur.

The prototype of endogenous hyperinsulinism with hypoglycemia is the β-cell tumor of the pancreatic islets (insulinoma). Although only 10% of such tumors metastasize, they are not infrequently multiple. Similar pathophysiology occurs in patients with β-cell hyperplasia or with a disorder termed nesidioblastosis, in which the islet cells are normal but additional duct-associated β-cells are scattered throughout the pancreas. Lastly, the rare patient with hyperinsulinism and hypoglycemia corrected by resection of the bulk of the pancreas, which is histologically normal despite extensive study, supports the concept of a syndrome of "functional" hyperinsulinism without an anatomic correlate.

Normally, the plasma glucose concentration is a tightly regulated variable. In contrast, serum insulin levels vary widely, depending in large part upon the plasma glucose level. After glucose

* The term "nonsuppressible insulin-like activity" has been applied to bioassayable insulin-like activity not obliterated by the addition of large quantities of insulin antiserum. This activity is similar in certain ways to the activity of somatomedins.

ingestion, serum insulin levels commonly rise as much as tenfold. On the other hand, as plasma glucose concentrations fall below 50 to 60 mg/100 ml, insulin secretion virtually ceases, and serum insulin concentrations fall to very low levels, often below the lower limit of sensitivity of some immunoassays. In view of the wide range of normal serum insulin levels, fewer than 50% of patients with insulinomas or related disorders are found to have absolute hyperinsulinism, i.e., serum insulin levels clearly higher than the levels seen under any circumstances in normal subjects.* The consistent biochemical abnormality in patients with insulinomas is relative hyperinsulinism, i.e., serum insulin levels inappropriately high for the simultaneously determined plasma glucose concentration, which demonstrate a failure of the abnormal β-cell tissue to turn off insulin secretion normally. Thus, the critical determinations are measurements of serum insulin concentrations at a time when the plasma glucose concentration is less than 50 mg/100 ml. Normally, the serum insulin concentration should be less than 5 μU/ml—often undetectable—whereas in patients with hypoglycemia due to hyperinsulinism, the serum insulin levels generally exceed 10 μU/ml during hypoglycemia and are often much higher. Since relative hyperinsulinism is the critical, decision-making determination in the diagnosis of insulinomas and related disorders, it should be apparent that a sensitive and precise insulin assay is essential. Furthermore, multiple insulin measurements in several serum samples are preferable to a single measurement.

It should be emphasized that plasma glucose levels of less than 50 mg/100 ml after 24 hours or more of fasting are not, in themselves, pathologic. These levels are seen in some overtly normal subjects, especially children and women, who do not exhibit relative hyperinsulinism.

Although not generally available, assays of serum proinsulin can be of value in the diagnosis of hyperinsulinism in the uncommon patient in whom relative hyperinsulinism with standard

* Often, although not invariably, absolute hyperinsulinism after a provocative stimulus, such as intravenous tolbutamide, can be demonstrated in such patients.

serum insulin measurements is not clear cut. Absolute (and fractional) proinsulin levels are generally elevated in patients with insulinomas.

In summary, when a thorough clinical evaluation, including the indicated laboratory studies, fails to demonstrate the cause of fasting hypoglycemia, hyperinsulinism should be suspected, and serum insulin levels should be measured during hypoglycemia. Many patients with insulinomas are regularly hypoglycemic after an overnight fast (some become hypoglycemic a few hours after eating) and serum insulin levels can be measured to establish the diagnosis. The absence of hypoglycemia after an overnight fast does not exclude the diagnosis of hyperinsulinism (as many as 20% of patients with insulinomas are said to have normal plasma glucose levels after an overnight fast), and a more prolonged fast may be required. As a general, and admittedly arbitrary, rule in patients in whom hyperinsulinism is suspected (on clinical grounds or because of the demonstration of frank, unexplained hypoglycemia in the past), but in whom the plasma glucose is greater than 50 mg/100 ml after an overnight fast, testing during a prolonged fast should be performed. Clearly, this must be performed in the hospital with the patient under competent supervision. The patient is permitted only calorie-free beverages, and the plasma glucose concentration is measured serially. Although a common recommendation is for sampling every 6 hours and whenever the patient has symptoms at all suggestive of hypoglycemia, in practice the sampling schedule should be individualized. (If the plasma glucose level is 55 mg/100 ml after an overnight fast it could be 25 mg/100 ml after six additional hours of fasting.) When the plasma glucose concentration is less than 50 mg/100 ml, an additional sample should be drawn to confirm the presence of hypoglycemia. Once the physician is convinced that fasting hypoglycemia has been demonstrated, the fast is terminated. Although it is common practice to measure serum insulin levels on all samples drawn during the fast, insulin measurements on the hypoglycemic samples are the critical determinations. In one large study, 96% of patients with hyperinsulinism developed hypoglycemia in less than 48 hours of fasting. Some investigators have taken the view that 72 hours of fasting without hypoglycemia is required to exclude the diagnosis.

The 72-hour fast is unpleasant for the patient, inconvenient for the hospital staff, and expensive. A better method to exclude the diagnosis is urgently needed, especially since the diagnosis of hyperinsulinism is often considered but infrequently made. A variety of short maneuvers have been proposed (such as the exaggerated insulin response and prolonged hypoglycemic response to intravenous tolbutamide), but in the author's judgment, the results of these maneuvers are not sufficiently distinctive to provide decision-making data. Thus, fasting hypoglycemia with relative hyperinsulinism must be demonstrated before surgery is recommended. After the decision to operate has been made, celiac arteriography is often performed, and it may be of particular value if metastases are demonstrated. A negative arteriogram, however, does not contraindicate pancreatic surgery if the clinical picture and biochemical data are convincing. A similar statement can be made about CT scans of the pancreas.

Reactive hypoglycemia (in the absence of fasting hypoglycemia) can be subdivided into three clinical categories:

1. Reactive hypoglycemia associated with mild diabetes mellitus.
2. "Alimentary" hypoglycemia.
3. Functional hypoglycemia.

Patients with elevated plasma glucose levels during the 1st 2 hours of a glucose tolerance test, who are hypoglycemic between the 3rd and 5th hours after oral glucose, are believed to have reactive hypoglycemia associated with diabetes mellitus. It has been suggested that delayed insulin release permits the development of hyperglycemia, ultimately eliciting a large insulin response, which, in turn, results in hypoglycemia in such patients; but this formulation is not universally accepted. "Alimentary" hypoglycemia is characterized by a rapid rise in the plasma glucose concentration to unusually high levels after oral glucose followed by hypoglycemia usually 90 to 180 minutes after ingestion. Early insulin levels are also quite high, and the hypoglycemia has been attributed to this. The results of intravenous glucose tolerance tests are generally normal in these patients. Alimentary hypoglycemia is most common in patients who have undergone gastric surgery, but this pattern of reactive hypoglycemia is now being recognized in patients with no history of gastrointestinal surgery and no recognizable gastrointestinal disease. The possibility that such patients overproduce insulin secretagogues of gastrointestinal origin in response to the ingestion of food has been raised. Perhaps the most common form of reactive hypoglycemia is the so-called functional hypoglycemia, in which the early portion of the plasma glucose curve following oral glucose is normal but hypoglycemia occurs between 2 and 4 hours after glucose ingestion. In these patients, serum insulin levels are not clearly distinguishable from normal, and the mechanism of the hypoglycemia is unknown.

Not only are the mechanisms of reactive hypoglycemia unclear, the definition of this disorder is a matter of some debate. Approximately 8% of nearly 5000 unselected, but overtly healthy, young adult men (military recruits) studied by Fariss had plasma glucose levels of less than 50 mg/100 ml 2 hours after a 100-gm oral glucose load (Fig. 9-3). If serial samples are obtained between 2 and 5 hours after oral glucose, an even greater proportion of apparently normal subjects are found to have glucose levels below 50 mg/100 ml. For example, in one study of 123 normal subjects, 23% were found to have one (or more) blood glucose level below 50 mg/100 ml (plasma glucose of approximately 58 mg/100 ml) 2 and 5 hours after oral glucose. Do such subjects have a "disease," which is apparently asymptomatic? Does recurrent asymptomatic hypoglycemia of this magnitude cause permanent damage? Does asymptomatic hypoglycemia progress to symptomatic hypoglycemia? The current judgment of some experts is that the answer to these questions is no. Perhaps, then, the arbitrary cutoff of less than 50 mg/100 ml is too high and should be revised downward, with normal values based on statistical evaluations of glucose tolerance tests from a large "normal" population. This might also fail to resolve the problem, however; although the data illus-

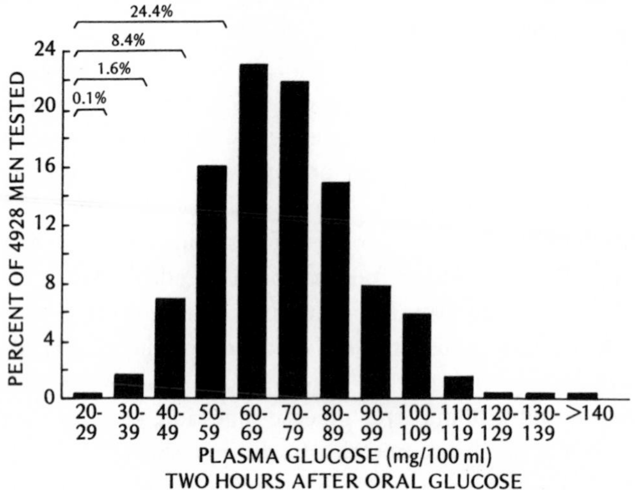

FIG. 9-3. Plasma glucose levels 2 hours after a 100-gm oral glucose load in 4928 overtly healthy, young, adult men. (From Fariss BL: *Diabetes* 23:189, 1974.)

trated in Fig. 9-3 suggest that a plasma glucose concentration of less than 40 mg/100 ml would be statistically abnormal, occasional patients with post-glucose plasma glucose concentrations between 30 and 40 mg/100 ml are apparently asymptomatic, whereas others with plasma glucose concentrations between 40 and 50 mg/100 ml are symptomatic. Thus, a reasonable clinical compromise is to diagnose reactive hypoglycemia only when a post-glucose plasma glucose concentration of less than 50 mg/100 ml is coupled temporally with symptoms consistent with hypoglycemia, which are alleviated with elevation of the plasma glucose concentration.

In summary, when reactive hypoglycemia is suspected, and fasting hypoglycemia can be confidently excluded, an oral glucose tolerance with frequent measurements of the plasma glucose concentration (preferably every 30 minutes) over at least 5 hours should be performed. During the test, the nature and time of occurrence of any symptoms noted by the patient should be recorded. In the author's judgment, the diagnosis of reactive hypoglycemia should be reserved for those patients with appropriate symptoms as well as biochemical hypoglycemia after a glucose load. Some would add a third criterion—a history of similar symptoms following meals—since oral glucose ingestion represents a non-physiologic stimulus. Certainly, such a history cannot be elicited in some patients with clinical and chemical reactive hypoglycemia during an oral glucose tolerance test.

SUGGESTED READING

1. Renold AE, Muller WA, Mintz DH, Cahill GF Jr: Diabetes mellitus. *In* The Metabolic Basis of Inherited Disease, Fourth Edition. Stanbury JB, Wyngaarden JB, Frederickson DS (eds). McGraw-Hill, New York, 1978, p 80.
2. Sussman KE, Metz RJS (eds): Diabetes mellitus, Fourth Edition. American Diabetes Association, New York, 1975.
3. Jarrett RJ, Keen H: Hyperglycemia and diabetes mellitus. *Lancet* 2:1009, 1976.
4. Gordon T, Castelli WP, Hjortland Mc, Kannel WB, Dawber TR: Diabetes, blood lipids and the role of obesity in coronary heart disease risk for women. *Ann Intern Med* 87:393, 1977.
5. Barbosa J, King R, Noreen H, Yunis EY: The histocompatibility system in juvenile, insulin dependent diabetic multiplex kindreds. *J Clin Invest* 60:989, 1977.
6. Fajans SS, Floyd JC Jr, Tattersal RB, Williamson JR, Pek S, Taylor CI: The various faces of diabetes in the young. *Arch Intern Med* 136:194, 1976.
7. Barbosa J, King R, Goetz FC, Noreen H, Yunis EJ: HLA in maturity-onset type of hyperglycemia in the young. *Arch Intern Med* 138:90, 1978.
8. Rubinstein P, Suciu-Foca N, Nicholson JF: Genetics of juvenile diabetes mellitus. *N Engl J Med* 297:1036, 1977.
9. Del Prete GF, Betterle C, Padovan D, Erle G, Toffolo A, Bershai G: Incidence and significance of islet cell autoantibodies in different types of diabetes mellitus. *Diabetes* 26:909, 1977.
10. Felig P, Wahren J, Sherwin R, Hendler R: Insulin, glucagon and somatostatin in normal physiology and diabetes mellitus. *Diabetes* 25:1091, 1976.
11. Kahn CR, Megyesi K, Bar RS, Eastman RC, Flier JS: Receptors for peptide hormones. *Ann Intern Med* 86:205, 1977.
12. Olefsky JM: The insulin receptor: Its role in insulin resistance of obesity and diabetes. *Diabetes* 25:1154, 1976.

13. Bunn HF, Gabbay KH, Gallop PM: The glycosylation of hemoglobin: Relevance to diabetes mellitus. *Science* 200:21, 1978.
14. Kreisberg RA: Diabetic ketoacidosis: New concepts and trends in pathogenesis and treatment. *Ann Intern Med* 88:681, 1978.
15. Marliss EB, Ohman JL, Aoki TT et al: Altered redox state obscuring ketoacidosis in patients with lactic acidosis. *N Engl J Med* 283: 978, 1970.
16. Arieff AI, Carroll HJ: Nonketotic hyperosmolar coma with hyperglycemia. *Medicine* 51:73, 1972.
17. Blankenship GW, Skylar JS: Diabetic retinopathy: A general survey. *Diabetes Care* 1:127, 1978.
18. Kussman MJ, Goldstein HH, Gleason RE: The clinical course of diabetic nephropathy. *J Amer Med Assoc* 236:1861, 1976.
19. Ellenberg M: Diabetic neuropathy: Clinical Aspects. *Metabolism* 25:1627, 1976.
20. Crall FV, Roberts WC: The extramural and intramural coronary arteries in juvenile mellitus. *Amer J Med* 64:221, 1978.
21. Permutt MA: Postprandial hypoglycemia. *Diabetes* 25:719, 1976.
22. Fajans SS, Floyd JC Jr: Fasting hypoglycemia in adults. *N Engl J Med* 294:766, 1976.
23. Pagliara AS, Karl IE, Haymond MW, Kipnis DM: Hypoglycemia in infancy and childhood. *J Pediatrics* 82:365 and 558, 1973.
24. Tischler AS, Dichter MA, Biales B, Greene LA: Neuroendocrine neoplasms and their cells of origin. *N Engl J Med* 296:919, 1977.
25. Scarlett JA, Mako ME, Rubenstein AH et al: Factitious hypoglycemia: Diagnosis by measurement of C-peptide immunoreactivity and insulin-binding antibodies. *N Engl J Med* 297:1029, 1977.
26. Megyesi K, Kahn CR, Roth J et al: Hypoglycemia in association with extra-pancreatic tumors: Demonstration of elevated plasma NSIHL-s by a new radioreceptor assay. *J Clin Endocrinol Metab* 38:931, 1974.
27. Garber AJ, Bier DM, Cryer PE, Pagliara AS: Hypoglycemia in compensated chronic renal insufficiency: Substrate limitation of gluconeogenesis. *Diabetes* 23:982, 1974.
28. Anderson JH Jr, Blackard WG, Goldman J, Rubenstein AH: Diabetes and hypoglycemia due to insulin antibodies. *Amer J Med* 64:868, 1978.
29. Service FJ, Dale AJD, Elveback LR, Jiang N-S: Insulinoma. Clinical and diagnostic features in 60 consecutive cases. *Mayo Clin Proc* 51:417, 1976.
30. Hirsch HJ, Loos S, Evans N, Crigler JF Jr, Filler RM, Gabbay KH: Hypoglycemia of infancy and nesidioblastosis. *N Engl J Med* 296:1323, 1977.

INDEX

Page numbers for figures and tables are in italics